Research Report

Navigating the Road to Reintegration

Status and Continuing Support of the U.S. Air Force's Wounded Warriors

Carra S. Sims, Christine Anne Vaughan, Haralambos Theologis, Ashley L. Boal, Karen Chan Osilla

RAND Project AIR FORCE

Prepared for the United States Air Force
Approved for public release; distribution unlimited

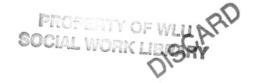

For more information on this publication, visit www.rand.org/t/RR599

Library of Congress Control Number: 2015943481

ISBN: 978-0-8330-8838-3

Published by the RAND Corporation, Santa Monica, Calif.

© Copyright 2015 RAND Corporation

RAND® is a registered trademark.

Support RAND
Make a tax-deductible charitable contribution at
www.rand.org/giving/contribute

www.rand.org

Preface

The United States has been at war for over a decade. As is inevitable, war imposes costs upon nations, not least of which is the cost to the nation's servicemembers. Although, comparatively speaking, the U.S. Air Force has suffered few casualties (Fischer, 2010), many airmen were injured in hostile or combat-related incidents. The Air Force wanted to understand the well-being of its members who were injured in combat, including their quality of life and the challenges that will confront them over the long term following separation or retirement. It was also interested in gauging the quality of support given to its veterans. The Air Force turned to RAND's Project AIR FORCE for help in assessing these areas of concern and requested an approach that would provide a foundation for a longitudinal exploration of the reintegration of its wounded warriors, with the ultimate goal being an ability to conduct such a longitudinal exploration. This report describes that baseline research effort.

The research reported here was commissioned by the Assistant Secretary of the Air Force for Manpower and Reserve Affairs (SAF/MR); the Director, Air Force Directorate of Services (AF/A1S); and the Air Force Surgeon General (AF/SG). The analysis was conducted within the Manpower, Personnel, and Training Program of RAND Project AIR FORCE as part of a fiscal year 2010–2012 project, "Tracking the Effectiveness of Warrior and Survivor Care." This report should interest those concerned with the status of the Air Force's wounded warriors and the quality of support they are receiving.

RAND Project AIR FORCE

RAND Project AIR FORCE (PAF), a division of the RAND Corporation, is the U.S. Air Force's federally funded research and development center for studies and analyses. PAF provides the Air Force with independent analyses of policy alternatives affecting the development, employment, combat readiness, and support of current and future air, space, and cyber forces. Research is performed in four programs: Force Modernization and Employment; Manpower, Personnel, and Training; Resource Management; and Strategy and Doctrine. The research reported here was prepared under contract FA7014-06-C-0001.

Additional information about PAF is available at:
http://www.rand.org/paf/

Contents

Preface.. iii

Figures... vii

Tables... ix

Summary... xi

Acknowledgments... xvii

Abbreviations... xix

1. Introduction.. 1
   Project Objectives... 1
   Analytical Approach.. 2
   Organization of the Report 3

2. Literature Review: A Holistic Approach to Reintegration Is Necessary...... 5
   Mental Health 7
      PTSD 7
      Depression 10
      Substance Use and Abuse... 12
      Consequences of Comorbid PTSD and Depression 13
   Physical Health 13
      Traumatic Brain Injury 13
   Other Relevant Domains of Functioning... 14
      Social Functioning and Interpersonal Relationships 14
      Unemployment and Financial Issues.. 16
      Housing Instability 20
   Opportunities for Intervention 22
      Mental and Physical Health.. 23
      Social Functioning and Interpersonal Relationships 25
      Unemployment and Financial Issues.. 25
      Housing Instability 26
   Summary... 27

3. Survey Method.. 29
   Sampling of Participants.. 29
   Procedure for Administering the Survey 30
   Measures Used in the Survey 31
      Sociodemographic and Service History Characteristics...................... 34

4. Survey Results 35
   Participants in the Survey 35

Mental Health and Substance Abuse 38
Physical Health and Medical Care...41
    Screening for Traumatic Brain Injury 41
    General Physical Health 42
Mental Health Services Utilization, Barriers, and Preferences 43
    Barriers to Treatment..46
    Preferred Setting 50
Interpersonal Relationships 54
Occupational Functioning..57
Financial Stability..62
Housing Instability...63
Program Evaluation 68
    Air Force Wounded Warrior Program...68
    Air Force Recovery Care Coordinator Program..70

5. Conclusions and Recommendations 75
Brief Caveats 76
Mental Health 78
    Inform Airmen About the Quality of Care Available to Them 78
    Emphasize and Enhance Confidential Treatment Options...81
    Seek Ways to Address Scheduling Difficulties...83
Employment...84
    Offered Employment Assistance Should Focus on Individual Skill Sets and Their
    Translation to New Contexts 85
    Reserve Component Members Need Continuing Attention...86
Conclusion 86

A. Detailed Measures Information..87

B. Survey Instrument 99

C. Additional Results 131

References 139

Figures

Figure 2.1. Holistic Model of Interrelationships and Intervention Opportunities 6

Figure 4.1. Positive Screens for PTSD and MDD, by Current Duty Status 40

Figure 4.2. Service Utilization and Need for Those Who Screened Positive for
PTSD or MDD 44

Figure 4.3. Receipt of Past-Year Mental Health Services, by Duty Status 45

Figure 4.4. Differences in Mental Health Treatment Barriers, by Current Duty
Status (N = 199) 49

Figure 4.5. Preferred Settings for Mental Health Treatment (N = 459) 52

Figure 4.6. Number of Different Residence Locations Within the Past Six Months........ 65

Figure 4.7. Housing Situation in Prior Six Months of Airmen with Lifetime
History of Homelessness.. 66

Tables

Table 3.1. Survey Measures Overview 32

Table 4.1. Respondent Characteristics (N = 459) 37

Table 4.2. Positive Screens for PTSD and MDD (N = 459) 38

Table 4.3. Rates of Alcohol and Illicit Drug Use in the Past 12 Months (N = 459) 41

Table 4.4. Positive Screens for Injuries and Possible TBI Sustained During
Deployment or Deployment-Related Activities (N = 459) 42

Table 4.5. Current Physical Health (N = 459) 43

Table 4.6. Medical Care Utilization and Desire and Health Insurance Status and
Need (N = 459) 43

Table 4.7. Barriers to Mental Health Services Utilization (N = 459) 47

Table 4.8. Mental Health Services Utilization in the Past 12 Months (N = 459) 49

Table 4.9. Mental Health Treatment Settings, by Current Duty Status (N = 459) 50

Table 4.10. Mental Health Services Preferences (N = 459) 51

Table 4.11. Final Multivariate Regression Model Predicting Civilian Provider
Preferences (N = 459) 54

Table 4.12. Current Relationship Status and Length of Current Relationship
(N = 459) 55

Table 4.13. Relationship of Primary Supporter to Airman (N = 459) 56

Table 4.14. Average Levels of Relationship Satisfaction with Marriage or
Relationship with Primary Supporter (N = 459) 57

Table 4.15. Current Employment Status (N = 459) 57

Table 4.16. Current Employment Status, Excluding Active Duty (N = 332) 59

Table 4.17. Job Performance and Satisfaction (N = 210) 60

Table 4.18. Perceived Barriers to Employment (N = 152) 61

Table 4.19. Financial Resources and Responsibilities 62

Table 4.20. Lifetime History of Homelessness (N = 459) 64

Table 4.21. Classification of Housing Situation Options 65

Table 4.22. Self-Reported Housing Situation During the Past Six Months of
Airmen with a Lifetime History of Potential Homelessness (N = 99) 67

Table 4.23. Housing Resources That Have Been Received or Would Be Helpful
(N = 459) 67

Table 4.24. Air Force Wounded Warrior Program Utilization (N = 459) 68

Table 4.25. Air Force Wounded Warrior Program Perceptions (N = 437) 69

Table 4.26. Air Force Recovery Care Coordinator Program Utilization (N = 459) 71

Table 4.27. Air Force Recovery Care Coordinator Program Services Utilized
(N = 91) 72

Table 4.28. Air Force Recovery Care Coordinator Program Perceptions (N = 91) 73

Table 4.29. Potential Concerns about AFRCC Services Utilization (N = 91) 73

Table C.1. Comparison of Medically Retired and Active-Duty Airmen Served
by the Air Force Wounded Warrior Program to Survey Completers
(N = 872) 131

Table C.2. Health Insurance Status (N = 459) 133

Table C.3. Specific Details on Mental Health Services (N = 459) 134

Table C.4. Number and Ages of Dependents 134

Table C.5. Household Structure (N = 459) 135

Table C.6. Perceived Social Support Available to Airman from Different People
in His/Her Life (N = 459) 135

Table C.7. Work Involvement (N = 459) 136

Table C.8. Financial Aid for Education and Job Training (N = 459) 136

Table C.9. Vocational Rehabilitation Services Utilization (N = 459) 137

Summary

The United States has been fighting wars in Iraq and then Afghanistan for well over a decade. Those conflicts have exacted a toll, not only in treasure and blood but also on servicemembers who have returned from the battlefield with physical and mental injuries and illnesses. Some remain on active duty, some move into the reserves, and others leave the service and seek civilian employment. However, all face a range of challenges, from reestablishing patterns of everyday interactions with their families to finding a job. Many must also cope with injuries and the treatment for those wounds. They must seek mental health services in some cases or navigate the complex array of the programs and systems of care available to veterans. The military services and the Department of Veterans Affairs have aggressively developed programs to help servicemembers reintegrate, with particular interest in mitigating the difficulties of reintegration for servicemembers with mental wounds. The U.S. Air Force wanted to gain greater insight into the well-being of its members who have sustained mental or physical injuries in combat or combat-related situations, with an eye toward improving services provided and enabling wounded airmen to become fully functioning members of society, and taking advantage of ongoing research into how best to do so. Areas of interest include their quality of life and the challenges that will impede their reintegration following separation or retirement. To begin the process of gaining this insight, the Air Force asked RAND's Project AIR FORCE for assistance in gauging the current status of the Air Force's wounded warriors, including their use of and satisfaction with Air Force programs designed to serve them. This report presents the baseline findings from the longitudinal analysis undertaken to understand these ongoing issues.

How We Went About the Analysis

Understanding the quality of life and challenges facing wounded warriors is a multifaceted task. We reviewed the history of physical, psychological, personal, and social adjustment difficulties experienced by veterans of previous wars, which emphasized the need to examine reintegration from a holistic perspective. Within the broad categories of difficulties discussed in the literature, we focused on four primary domains: mental health, unemployment, homelessness, and interpersonal relationships. Each domain is a potential target of interventions and policies that the Air Force could implement. By focusing on these domains, we present a relatively comprehensive picture of the reintegration of returning wounded warriors and help answer the Institute of Medicine's (2010) call for a more complex and holistic examination of reintegration.

To assess these domains throughout the process of reintegration, we fielded a survey to serve as the baseline assessment in a longitudinal analysis of the lives of airmen who sustained mental or physical wounds in combat or combat-related situations. According to the Air Force's administrative data, the majority of airmen in the sampling frame (74 percent) had received a diagnosis of post-traumatic stress disorder (PTSD). Thus, mental health was identified as a key reintegration challenge for the airmen in our sample before the survey's development. Guided by the literature, we included validated measures for assessing the presence of various psychological disorders, barriers to employment and job satisfaction, indicators of housing instability, and some established measures of other domains. The survey also asked respondents to evaluate the care and service they have received from the Air Force, specifically the Air Force Wounded Warrior (AFW2) program and the Air Force Recovery Care Coordinator (AFRCC) program. The AFW2 program coordinates services other than medical care for airmen injured in combat or activities related to combat (this may include deployment-related training). The AFRCC program employs Recovery Care Coordinators whose purpose is to ensure recovering airmen and families understand the likely recovery path, oversee the development and implementation of airmen's Comprehensive Recovery Plans, work with Medical Care Case Managers, and advocate for airmen. We fielded this survey in the fall of 2011 to the enrollees in the Air Force Wounded Warriors Program who were receiving benefits or undergoing evaluation to receive benefits. This approach enabled us to reach our target population: Airmen who have typically suffered injuries in combat or related situations that had either caused them to retire or were considered likely to cause them to retire or separate from the military.[1] Thus, our holistic approach is applied to a highly selected and unique population of airmen who have been identified as having injuries and illnesses that are related to combat and who are particularly vulnerable to suffering long-term effects from their wounds.

Using the AFW2 enrollee census enabled us to identify reliable locations of retirees, whose current contact information would otherwise not be contained in Air Force personnel files. This approach enabled us to incorporate former airmen who otherwise might be difficult to contact. Of the 872 airmen who were invited to participate, 493 started the survey; the majority of these, 459 (for an overall response rate of 53 percent), completed it either over the web or by phone. These airmen largely resembled the broader population of wounded retirees and active-duty airmen enrolled in AFW2, with some minor differences in that they were slightly more likely to have a college degree, were about a year older, and had spent about a year longer on active duty. The majority

---

[1] Note that some do in fact remain in service rather than separating or retiring.

of respondents, like the population itself, were retired, male, and white; and most were former enlisted servicemembers.

Results in Brief

Our results show that airmen in our sample are indeed experiencing challenges in a number of different domains. Our results, which parallel those of the Air Force, show a high proportion of airmen screening positive for current PTSD (roughly 78 percent) and current major depressive disorder (MDD) (roughly 75 percent), with 69 percent screening positive for both. We also find somewhat elevated rates of reported substance use over the past year relative to the U.S. adult general population and low levels of current self-rated physical heath relative to a civilian sample of adults with physical and mental chronic illnesses. Although the current sample reported very high rates of mental health treatment within the past year for those who screened positive for current PTSD or current MDD (90 percent), within that same time frame about half indicated there was at least one instance when they desired mental health treatment but did not receive it. A one-year time frame is broad. However, given the identified need for mental health services among this population and the efforts that have been undertaken to better address servicemembers' mental health needs, failure to receive treatment when desired remains a pertinent issue.

Reported barriers to receiving mental health care reveal ongoing concerns regarding confidentiality and stigma, though the current data do not link these concerns to a particular treatment setting (i.e., civilian, medical treatment facility, or Veterans Affairs). Other concerns regarding the quality of available treatment are also evident and included the belief that available mental health treatments are not very good and concerns about the side effects of psychotropic medication. A reported preference for civilian providers is potentially troubling because of findings that civilian mental health care is not likely to be driven by an evidence base (e.g., Institute of Medicine, 2006; President's New Freedom Commission on Mental Health, 2003).

Survey responses also suggested potential deficits in social support among airmen. Airmen were asked to identify the nature of their relationship to the one individual "who most often helps you deal with problems that come up," i.e., their "primary supporter." Nearly one-half of respondents selected their spouse or domestic partner as their primary supporter. Minorities of respondents (i.e., less than 10 percent) named a friend, parent or parent-in-law, other relative, or boyfriend or girlfriend as their primary supporter. Just over one-quarter of respondents indicated that they did not have a primary supporter, i.e., they did not share their problems with anyone. Not having an identified primary supporter may be because of a dearth of social support resources or personal choice not to share problems. Hence, the proportion reporting this status may or may not consider it a problem that they do not have someone with whom to share. Nonetheless, it may be considered an indicator of potential risk in terms of availability of social support resources.

Findings in other domains also reveal vulnerabilities. Although a comparatively low proportion of airmen reported falling below the U.S. Department of Health and Human Services' poverty guidelines, about 10 percent could be considered as living in poverty. Similarly, close to 15 percent would be considered unemployed based on the U.S. Bureau of Labor Statistics' oft-reported U3 measure of unemployment. High unemployment rates are common in the current economic situation, but these rates may represent a particular concern for our population. Moreover, some of the perceived barriers to employment suggest interventions in the form of skills training and provision of jobs information would be beneficial. For example, some respondents felt concern regarding their qualifications, in particular that their deployments put them behind their civilian counterparts (42 percent) or a general lack of confidence (42 percent).

Housing instability represents another potential area of concern, with almost 10 percent of the entire sample indicating that their first experience with potential homelessness occurred after their return from their most recent deployment. Further analysis showed that relatively few airmen were homeless; that said, given the well-known troubles of past generations of veterans, this domain warrants continued attention.

Across the domains examined, Reserve and Guard members evidenced heightened challenges. They indicated more severe symptoms of mental health disorders and subsequently met screening criteria for mental health diagnoses at a higher rate than active component airmen still on active duty. Within the domain of employment, Reserve and Guard personnel who indicated that they were employed at least part time also indicated that their productivity was lower than did our other duty status groups.

Finally, we also asked questions regarding use of and satisfaction with two Air Force programs available to help these airmen. High numbers of respondents indicated that they were receiving services, particularly from the AFW2 program. This is a positive finding because our population consisted of enrollees in that program. Respondents also reported overall satisfaction with the program. Although eligibility requirements dictated that a smaller proportion of our population would be covered by the AFRCC program, airmen who reported receipt of AFRCC services received a variety of them and were very satisfied with the program. For both programs, the nature of services provided can be characterized as a form of social support.

Policy Recommendations and Conclusions

We focus our recommendations on two domains: mental health and employment. We do so because the problems in these domains were notably elevated and amenable to intervention. We also focus on areas where Air Force case managers could take action. Finally, concerns in these areas, if mitigated, would be expected to have a positive influence on problems in other domains.[2]

Mental Health Recommendations

Our recommendations in the mental health domain are designed to deal with the reported barriers to accessing mental health services. To overcome these barriers to treatment, we recommend that the Air Force (and other related systems of care) take the following actions to increase airmen's receipt of high-quality mental health treatment:

- Inform airmen about the quality of care available to them.
  - Collect and publicize data on the quality of care that is implemented.
  - Educate airmen on the questions to ask prospective mental health care providers to improve their chances of getting high-quality treatment.
  - Inform airmen on the options for psychotropic medications and alternatives to them.
- Emphasize and enhance confidential treatment options.
  - Promote available confidential nonmedical counseling options for airmen who would otherwise forgo mental health treatment.
  - Place mental health care providers in primary care clinics.

Employment Recommendations

The employment literature suggests that attention to individual skill sets and their presentation on resumes and in interviews, as well as individual preferences, pay dividends in the forms of employment, lasting employment, and satisfaction (Drake, Bond, and Becker, 2012; Resnick, Rosenheck, and Drebing, 2006; Wanberg, 2012). Our recommendations capitalize on both this finding and the existence of the many employment aid offerings already provided for wounded, ill, and injured warriors (GAO, 2012, noted 19 different programs in FY 2010). We do not recommend additional programs but rather suggest that the employment assistance to airmen should focus on individual skill sets and their translation to new contexts.

To help those who are unemployed, we recommend the following actions:

- Offer employment assistance that focuses on individual skill sets and their transition to new contexts; continue existing programs that have this individual focus.
- Identify and continue to treat mental health disorders.

---

[2] For example, improving employment outcomes would likely promote housing stability.

Our findings regarding the multidomain challenges experienced by Reserve and Guard servicemembers in our sample in tandem with the larger literature indicate the Reserve and Guard may be more vulnerable to various issues. These include experiencing heightened PTSD symptoms postdeployment (e.g., Schell and Marshall, 2008; Wells et al., 2011) and suggest continued attention to the needs of the reserve components will be necessary to make sure the care they receive meets their needs. The process of recovery and reintegration is likely to be lengthy, particularly for those with injuries and illnesses. A long-term approach is needed to parse the effectiveness of the many interventions and conditions that affect it. Thus, we suggest ongoing program evaluation. Many studies have examined various aspects of the reintegration problem, but much remains to be done. Moreover, because no one study can encompass the complexities of real life, it is appropriate to take advantage of quality research from multiple avenues. The Air Force, by means of this research project and others, is starting to compile the information it needs to understand the process of recovery and reintegration. Our data are cross-sectional. We therefore present a snapshot of wounded airmen's well-being on a holistic set of indicators. Our findings reveal that enrollees in the AFW2 program are facing a variety of reintegration challenges. These are likely to remain pressing. The Air Force and society at large must continue to provide support through this process. In a time of declining resources, research can help determine the most effective means to do so.

Acknowledgments

We have many people to thank for contributing to this multiyear project. We would like to begin by thanking our research commissioners, Daniel Ginsberg, Brigadier General Eden J. Murrie, and Lieutenant General (Dr.) Thomas W. Travis. We would also like to thank John Beckett, the first action officer for the project, whose concern for the Air Force and its wounded warriors got the project off on the right foot. The continued support of our other action officers, Edmundo Gonzales, Lieutenant Colonel Michael Wyatt, and Colonel Todd Poindexter, helped make the project's completion possible. They tirelessly offered guidance and support. We would also like to thank Tim Townes and Major Nicole Fuller.

Many others offered their experienced perspective to enable this study. These include Lieutenant Colonel David Bringhurst, Lieutenant Colonel Susan Black, and Marsha Gonzales, of the AFW2 program, who shared with us their experience with the Air Force's wounded warriors. We would also like to thank Stephen Page and the Air Force Recovery Care Coordinators who spoke with us about their experiences as case managers, as well as the AFW2 case managers who spoke with us and offered advice and perspective along the way.

We also thank the three reviewers who read our document carefully and offered many suggestions to make this a stronger and more readable work; Jerry Sollinger, who tried to keep us on track in terms of clarity of expression; and Jamie Greenberg, who provided administrative support.

Most of all we thank the wounded warriors who took the time to answer our questions and offer insight into their current status.

Abbreviations

AF/A1S	Air Force Directorate of Services
AF/SG	Air Force Surgeon General
AFPC	Air Force Personnel Center
AFRCC	Air Force Recovery Care Coordinator Program
AFW2	Air Force Wounded Warrior Program
AUD	alcohol use disorder
AUDIT-C	Alcohol Use Disorders Identification Test—Consumption
BLS	Bureau of Labor Statistics
BTBIS	Brief Traumatic Brain Injury Scale
CBT	cognitive behavioral therapy
CI	confidence interval
CPT	cognitive processing therapy
CRP	Comprehensive Recovery Plan
DES	Disability Evaluation System
DoD	Department of Defense
DSM-IV	Diagnostic and Statistical Manual of Mental Disorders, Fourth Edition
DSM-IV-TR	Diagnostic and Statistical Manual of Mental Disorders
EBT	evidence-based treatment
EMDR	eye movement desensitization and reprocessing
HHS	Department of Health and Human Services
HUD-VASH	U.S. Department of Housing and Urban Development–Veterans Affairs Supported Housing
IED	improvised explosive device
IOM	Institute of Medicine
IPT	interpersonal therapy
LOC	loss of consciousness
MDD	major depressive disorder
MFLC	Military and Family Life Counselor
MOU	memorandum of understanding
MTF	military treatment facility
NIMH	National Institute of Mental Health
NESARC	National Epidemiologic Survey on Alcohol and Related Conditions
OEF	Operation Enduring Freedom

OIF	Operation Iraqi Freedom
OR	odds ratio
PAF	Project AIR FORCE
PCL	PTSD checklist
PE	prolonged exposure
PTSD	post-traumatic stress disorder
RCC	Recovery Care Coordinator
RCP	Recovery Care Plan
SAF/MR	Secretary of the Air Force for Manpower and Reserve Affairs
SD	standard deviation
SF-36	Short Form health survey with 36 questions
SPS	Social Provisions Scale
SI	seriously injured
SSRI	selective serotonin reuptake inhibitor
TBI	traumatic brain injury
UL	upper limit
VA	Veterans Affairs
VASH	Veterans Affairs Supported Housing
VHA	Veterans Health Administration
VISN	Veterans Integrated Service Network
VSI	very seriously injured

1. Introduction

Comparatively speaking, the United States Air Force has suffered few casualties over more than a decade of war (Fischer, 2010). However, many airmen were injured in hostile or combat-related incidents. The Air Force wanted to understand the well-being of its members, current and former, who have sustained combat injuries. It wanted to get a sense of their quality of life and the challenges that impede their reintegration into society over the long term. The Air Force turned to RAND's Project AIR FORCE for help in assessing these areas of concern and requested an analysis that would provide a foundation for a longitudinal exploration of the reintegration of their wounded warriors.

Project Objectives

When this project originated, its goals included seeking a broad perspective on the numerous challenges that accompany reintegration. The contingency operations of the last decade differed from those of the past. Specifically, they depended heavily on the Reserve and Guard and saw an increase in the number, duration, and pace of deployments (Institute of Medicine [IOM], 2010). They have also lasted longer than any U.S. military operation. The warfare differs as well, with a more consistent focus on counterinsurgency and, in some cases, services such as the Navy and Air Force being employed in ground roles. Moreover, the advances made by medical science have enabled many to survive injuries that in previous conflicts would have proven fatal (Tanielian and Jaycox, 2008; Warden, 2006). The enduring consequences of the Vietnam War suggest that the challenges the nation currently faces are likely to persist. However, the differences in the nature of the conflict suggest that the course of reintegration and healing may raise more or different issues as these veterans reintegrate into society.

Existing research on reintegration has been more broadly focused on the needs of veterans across the spectrum of combat-related impairment. Although it is recognized that the psychosocial needs of veterans with combat injuries are greater in number and magnitude than the needs of those who do not have such injuries, an in-depth and holistic assessment of the needs of this particular subgroup of veterans has not yet been conducted. The current project is designed to fill this gap in the literature, using a longitudinal design. The initial desire for a broad perspective drove a holistic orientation and opened the door to consideration of numerous domains. Thus, we developed a notional model to orient and guide us in selection of psychosocial domains to consider and assess over the longitudinal course of reintegration. This report presents the findings from the baseline survey. Future work would consider this baseline and improve upon it, driven by questions sparked by this initial survey as well as by the changing needs of the Air Force and its wounded warriors.

Analytical Approach

The Air Force has two main programs that serve its wounded warriors: The Air Force Wounded Warrior (AFW2) program and the Air Force Recovery Care Coordinator (AFRCC) program. During the study period, the AFW2 coordinated services other than medical care for airmen injured in combat or activities related to combat (this may include deployment-related training).[1] According to Air Force Instruction (AFI) 34-1101 (2012), which codified many of the processes informally in place at the time of study inception, the program connects recovering airmen and families with resources and services to solve problems that are nonmedical in nature throughout the continuum of care (p.18). The AFRCC program employs Recovery Care Coordinators whose purpose is to ensure recovering airmen and families understand the likely recovery path, to oversee the development and implementation of airmen's Comprehensive Recovery Plans, to work with Medical Care Case Managers, and to advocate for airmen (p. 27). The AFRCC program serves a more severely injured subset of the combat-injured airmen who are enrolled in the AFW2 program and airmen whose injuries are not combat related.

Airmen who were enrollees in the AFW2 program during our study period had typically suffered injuries such that they had either medically separated or retired from the military or were seen as likely to do so. Although deployment can have negative consequences even without grievous psychological or physical injuries, the Air Force asked Project AIR FORCE to focus on AFW2 enrollees. Given that our population of interest is those with recognized combat-related injuries severe enough to warrant consideration for medical retirement, we expect that the prevalence and severity of psychosocial challenges documented in previous research will be amplified in our sample compared with those with less severe injuries and illnesses.

Additionally, our sample is specifically restricted to airmen whose experiences may differ qualitatively from those of other servicemembers, although all are indubitably subject to trauma. Within the broader context of psychosocial functioning, we consider the four primary domains of mental health, unemployment, homelessness, and interpersonal relationships. Each domain is suggested by the literature as important.

---

[1] This was initiated in 2005 and known as Air Force Palace HART (Helping Airmen Recover Together); it was renamed in 2007 as the Air Force Wounded Warrior Program (Grill, 2012). Note that some changes in the conduct of programs for seriously ill and injured airmen, as well as those with combat-related injuries, have taken place through 2012, including expansion of eligibility criteria.

Moreover, each is a potential target for interventions and policies that the Air Force could implement, and we provide information on the evidence base that supports their use. The domains of mental health and employment are particularly amenable to intervention, given the relatively robust evidence base upon which to rest recommendations. In addition, intervening in the areas of mental health and employment may prevent later negative spillover into other domains, although causality may ultimately be reciprocal.

Based on our purview and the literature documenting some of the challenges experienced by veterans of the Vietnam War and known concerns of the current conflicts, we developed a notional model that drove a survey that assessed well-being on a number of critical indicators. These indicators included psychological health, social support, housing instability, and perceived financial security. We also included questions to assess Air Force services used, focusing on the AFW2 program and the AFRCC program. As the programs were established relatively recently, no formal evaluations of how well they meet the needs of combat-injured medically separated and retired airmen have been conducted yet. Program evaluation is critical for both accountability and program improvement. Specific goals of program evaluation are to determine the array and extent of the needs of intended program recipients, assess how well the program meets these needs, and provide guidance for program improvement. Thus, this analysis provides an independent evaluation and an important resource for the Air Force in determining how best to meet the needs of Air Force wounded warriors.

Organization of the Report

In Chapter Two, we describe the model we developed and review the literature documenting challenges that reintegration is likely to entail, taking a holistic perspective that considers several domains of functioning as described earlier. In Chapter Three, we provide an overview of our survey procedure and content that are driven by the literature and our notional model. In Chapter Four, we detail the results of the baseline survey itself. Finally, in Chapter Five, we describe the conclusions we drew from this baseline investigation and provide recommendations for the Air Force to consider based on our findings and the wider literature.

2. Literature Review: A Holistic Approach to Reintegration Is Necessary

In assessing individuals with reintegration challenges potentially exacerbated by their injuries, several life domains warrant consideration. A holistic perspective suggests that the nature of the injury itself is important and that social and work functioning as well as other stressors, such as housing instability, should be included (see, e.g., Berglass and Harrell, 2012; IOM, 2010). The purpose of the current project was to lay a foundation for a longitudinal effort. Thus, we surveyed the literature with the goal of determining what functional domains should be included in this holistic perspective. We then developed a notional model that guided our selection of variables for a baseline survey, the results of which are also presented in this report.

Our notional holistic model is portrayed in Figure 2.1. The variables include health, particularly post-traumatic stress disorder (PTSD) and depression; social support; housing status; and job and financial status—all of which are expected to influence each other. As shown, we also include the provision of services, which are hoped to influence each of these variable sets in ways that benefit the overall reintegration of wounded warriors. Ultimately, all of these variables are of interest because of their potential effect upon the process of reintegration; but the provision of services represents the hope that policy decisionmakers may be able to mitigate some of the challenges faced by those who have given much in service to the country. The bi-directionality of all of the arrows in the figure demonstrates the interplay among the variable sets. The arrows from services are black to indicate that these represent the effects of policy intervention. Although we include social support as a separate domain, reintegration programs such as the AFW2 program and the AFRCC program may themselves help mimic the natural support system (family, friends, community) during a time when the social supports are likely to be disrupted. Telephone calls and frequent contact with servicemembers allow these service providers—called "nonmedical case managers"—to advise, guide and assist with formulating life and recovery goals, or just listen.[1] Later, we discuss the literature that guided our selection of these areas for our holistic model and ultimately describe what interventions may be available to policymakers.

---

[1] We thank the reviewer who suggested this phrasing.

Figure 2.1. Holistic Model of Interrelationships and Intervention Opportunities

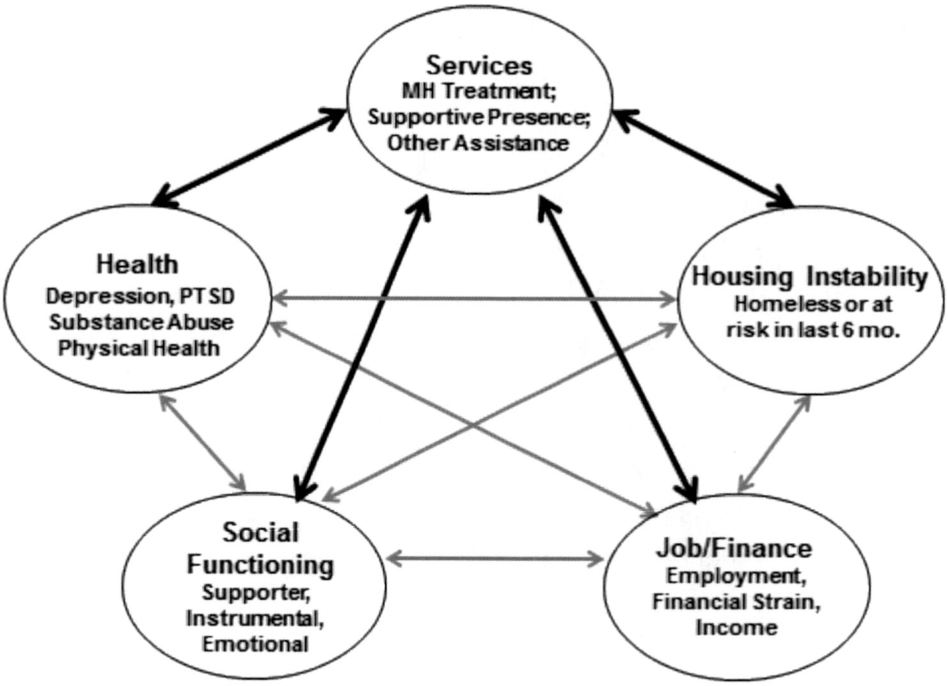

NOTE: MH = mental health; PTSD = post-traumatic stress disorder; mo. = months.

Given that the nature of the injury plays a key role, we first consider some of the injuries that have come to characterize the conflicts in Iraq and Afghanistan. We describe their nature and consider the information about their etiology and course. The work to date has often focused on general servicemember populations, to include soldiers, marines, and sailors, and airmen. Although some work examines individuals who are seeking care for concerns such as PTSD, much focuses more generally on servicemembers who have been deployed. However, the literature is nonetheless particularly relevant for the Air Force, because the primary injury of enrollees noted by the Air Force Wounded Warrior Program is PTSD. These airmen are a select and unique subset of the larger population of servicemembers who must chart the path of reintegration.[2] Their injuries, of course, neither occur nor heal in isolation. However, our focus is not primarily medical. Therefore we also consider interpersonal relationships and social functioning as well as functioning in a number of life domains such as housing stability, employment, and financial stability. These, in tandem with program initiatives to help these injured airmen, help present an overall picture of well-being and risk. We

---

[2] Note that although our study focuses on airmen, the general population and general veteran literature is relevant, particularly as relatively few studies focus exclusively on airmen.

first define the issues and then outline some available remedies, all of which informed our contextual understanding and helped to dictate what we included in the baseline survey for our longitudinal study.

Mental Health

Past research has demonstrated that rates of current probable PTSD and major depressive disorder (MDD) among servicemembers and veterans deployed in Operations Enduring Freedom and Iraqi Freedom (OEF/OIF) are notably elevated relative to those documented in the U.S. general population of adults (Hoge, 2004; Ramchand et al., 2010; Schell and Marshall, 2008; Vaughan et al., 2011). The noted frequency of PTSD among AFW2 program enrollees means that mental health problems represent a critical quality of life issue in the specific population of severely combat-wounded airmen enrolled.

Mental health conditions often co-occur with other problems such as substance use. In one study of new users in the Department of Veterans Affairs (VA) system, Alcohol Use Disorder (AUD) and comorbid mental health diagnoses were 3 to 4.5 times more likely in veterans with PTSD and depression (Seal et al., 2011). In another study of recently deployed National Guard members, participants who had PTSD or MDD were 17 to 22 percent more likely to develop alcohol use disorders after deployment (Grant et al., 2012). Participants were almost 50 percent more likely to develop alcohol use disorders after deployment if they had both PTSD and MDD. Thus, we briefly consider substance use as well.

In the following sections, we define relevant mental health conditions and discuss their etiology and prevalence. Subsequently we discuss applicable policy concerns and potential remedies.

PTSD

According to the Diagnostic and Statistical Manual of Mental Disorders, Fourth Edition Text Revision (DSM-IV-TR) definition,[3] PTSD is a constellation of symptoms that develop in response to a traumatic event (American Psychiatric Association, 2001). By this definition, a traumatic event is one in which an individual experienced or observed an event that involved actual or threatened physical harm to oneself or others and prompted intense fear, helplessness, or horror. The constellation of symptoms is

---

[3]   Note that the new DSM-5 definition of PTSD, introduced in 2013, is slightly different. Criteria include additional symptoms and establish four symptom clusters that distinguish active avoidance from negative alterations in cognitions and mood (DSM-IV criterion C symptoms) (see, e.g., Friedman et al., 2011). However, existing validated measures are keyed to the DSM-IV because our baseline survey was fielded prior to the release of the DSM-5.

organized into the following three clusters: re-experiencing of the event (e.g., repeated, disturbing memories of the event), avoidance of reminders of the event and numbing (e.g., efforts to avoid reminders of the trauma, diminished interest or involvement in activities that were of interest before the trauma), and hyperarousal (e.g., hypervigilance, problems sleeping) (American Psychiatric Association, 2001).

Most adults in the U.S. general population experience at least one potentially traumatic event in their lifetime (Kessler et al., 1995). However, most individuals who experience traumatic events do not subsequently develop PTSD (Bonanno, 2004, 2005). That is, the typical trajectory of PTSD symptoms experienced following a traumatic event is one of resilience. Estimates of the prevalence of PTSD in servicemembers and veterans who have deployed to OEF/OIF vary widely across studies (IOM, 2012; Ramchand et al., 2010). In a review of studies of the prevalence of current PTSD in samples of servicemembers previously deployed to Iraq or Afghanistan (Ramchand et al., 2010), estimates of PTSD ranged from roughly 5 to 20 percent. The variability of estimates from different studies primarily results from differences in the samples studied and the cutpoints applied to different screening instruments.

Little research has focused specifically on PTSD among airmen. One of the few exceptions, the Millennium Cohort Study, compared rates of new-onset PTSD across airmen who had deployed to Iraq or Afghanistan after 2001 to rates for those who had not deployed (Smith et al., 2008). Airmen who had deployed with combat exposure had rates of PTSD (3.5 percent) that were nearly three times as high as those who had not deployed during the same period (1.2 percent), after adjusting for several demographic and service history characteristics. Of note, these rates were roughly one-third of those reported by soldiers in the Millennium Cohort Study (9.3 percent of soldiers who deployed and had combat exposure had new-onset PTSD; 3 percent of soldiers who did not deploy had new-onset PTSD). Similarly, in another study of previously deployed OEF/OIF servicemembers, airmen had a lower risk of probable PTSD relative to soldiers in both unadjusted and adjusted models (Schell and Marshall, 2008). Thus, rates of PTSD among airmen appear to be low relative to those documented among soldiers, most likely owing to the fact that soldiers play a greater role in "boots on the ground" combat in which they are more likely to be exposed to traumatic events. Attributable largely to combat trauma, the risk of PTSD is significantly higher among previously deployed OEF/OIF servicemembers relative to their demographically similar peers in the U.S. general population (Hoge, 2004; Ramchand et al., 2010; Schell and Marshall, 2008; Vaughan et al., 2011). Combat exposure is the most robustly documented risk factor for PTSD among previously deployed OEF/OIF servicemembers and veterans (Ramchand et al., 2010). Several other risk factors have been identified in research on civilians and veterans. These include younger age at the time of the trauma (Brewin, Andrews, and Valentine, 2000), lack of education (Brewin et al., 2000), enlisted rank (Lapierre, Schwegler, and

LaBauve, 2007; Maguen et al., 2010; Schell and Marshall, 2008; Smith et al., 2008), black or Hispanic race/ethnicity (Brewin et al., 2000); military sexual trauma (Suris and Lind, 2008); and lack of social support (Brewin, Andrews, and Valentine, 2000; Ozer et al., 2003). Note that these risk factors tend to indicate that servicemembers have fewer resources and thus higher vulnerability to a variety of challenges, not just PTSD (e.g., see discussion in Tanielian and Jaycox, 2008).

The course of PTSD is, typically, one of declining symptom severity over time in studies of civilian samples (e.g., Blanchard et al., 1995; Schell, Marshall, and Jaycox, 2004). Similarly, based on a reanalysis of data from the National Vietnam Veterans Readjustment Study (NVVRS), it appears that "the trajectory for most veterans with war-related PTSD that causes substantial impairment is toward amelioration or complete remission" (Dohrenwend et al., 2006; p. 982); 18.7 percent of the Vietnam veterans in this sample had war-related PTSD during their lifetimes, and 9.1 percent of veterans met criteria for current PTSD 11 to 12 years following the Vietnam War. These findings contrast with those from longitudinal research on Gulf War veterans in which increases in PTSD rates (Wolfe et al., 1999) and symptoms (Southwick et al., 1995) were found during the two-year period following redeployment. However, these studies of Gulf War veterans followed veterans over a shorter period of time after the war than did the NVVRS; thus, differences in study findings may stem from differences in the studies' follow-up intervals.

Little is known about the course of PTSD symptoms among OEF/OIF veterans during reintegration into civilian society (Sundin et al., 2010). Two longitudinal studies of OEF/OIF veterans indicate that PTSD symptoms may worsen in the first few months following return from deployment (Bliese et al., 2007; Milliken et al., 2007). Similarly, increases in rates of probable PTSD between assessments conducted at three and 12 months following return from deployment to Iraq were found among the same four Active Component and two National Guard infantry Brigade Combat Teams (BCTs) (Thomas et al., 2010). However, in a longitudinal study that tracked UK veterans of the wars in Iraq and Afghanistan over a three-year period following deployment, 66 percent of respondents who screened positive for PTSD (as indicated by a score of 50 or more on the PTSD Checklist) at baseline reported symptoms consistent with partial or full remission at follow-up (Rona et al., 2012).

As the two aforementioned longitudinal studies on OEF/OIF servicemembers from the United States used data collected immediately after redeployment as the baseline (Bliese et al., 2007; Milliken et al., 2007), the observed increases in positive PTSD screens may be partly attributable to the timing of the PTSD assessment with respect to the servicemember's return from deployment. That is, servicemembers who report symptoms in an "on-the-record" screening immediately after returning from deployment may be inclined to underreport to avoid negative consequences of reporting, such as

9

incurring a delay in reuniting with their families. Consistent with this notion, in research comparing "on-the-record" assessments of mental health symptoms with anonymous assessments, higher rates of mental health problems have been documented in anonymous assessments (Warner et al., 2011). Thus, studies that use data collected from "on-the-record" screenings conducted immediately following deployment may underestimate the true rate of probable PTSD. Alternatively, the increases in PTSD symptoms may reflect true increases in PTSD symptoms.

Rather than examining the average course of PTSD over a single group of individuals, some researchers have examined subgroups of veterans with different symptom trajectories. For example, in one longitudinal study of Gulf War veterans, two groups of veterans were identified based on their PTSD symptom trajectories: those who reported low initial levels of PTSD symptoms that didn't increase much over time and those who reported higher initial levels of PTSD symptoms that increased significantly over time (Orcutt, Erickson, and Wolfe, 2004). Thus, the course of PTSD appears to be somewhat variable across individuals, with some individuals more prone to developing chronic PTSD than others.

From a policy standpoint, PTSD among combat veterans is troubling in light of the toll it exacts and its adverse implications for veterans' reintegration into civilian life. In addition, PTSD itself has been associated with lower quality of life and functional impairment in multiple domains, including the social, occupational, and physical domains (Kessler et al., 2000; Olatunji, Cisler, and Tolin, 2007; Schnurr et al., 2006; Zatzick et al., 1997), as has MDD (Pyne et al., 1997; Rapaport et al., 2005).

Depression

Major depressive disorder (MDD) is a mood disorder that consists of several pervasive depressive symptoms that interfere with everyday life. More than a passing sadness that is common to everyone, MDD is a persistent constellation of symptoms that occur most of the day or nearly every day for at least a two-week period (American Psychiatric Association Task Force on DSM-IV, 2000).

Prevalence estimates of MDD vary across studies depending on, among other things, the definition of depression used and whether functional impairment was a requirement of the definition, as well as the timing of the assessment with respect to the servicemember's return from deployment. In one study of Army and Marine combat units that had returned from a deployment to Iraq and Afghanistan three or four months earlier, roughly 7 percent of servicemembers met criteria for probable depression under a more stringent definition that required functional impairment, and roughly 15 percent met criteria under a less stringent definition that did not require functional impairment (Hoge et al., 2004). In another study, estimates of the prevalence of probable MDD with serious functional impairment among Active Component and National Guard soldiers one year after returning from a combat deployment to Iraq were 8.5 percent and 7.3 percent, respectively, and roughly 16 percent for both groups when the definition did not require functional impairment (Thomas et al., 2010). Other studies of formerly deployed OEF/OIF personnel in which probable MDD was assessed without consideration of functional impairment found that roughly 14 percent (Schell and Marshall, 2008) and 16 percent (Vaughan et al., 2011) of respondents met criteria for probable MDD. It is important to note that rates of depression, and other types of psychopathology more broadly, tend to be greater among individuals with a history of combat trauma exposure (e.g., Schell and Marshall, 2008) and so are unlikely to generalize to the force as a whole.

In addition, similar to PTSD, rates of depression may vary across studies because of differences in the timing of assessment with respect to the servicemember's return from deployment. For example, in one study, rates of probable depression among soldiers returning from a deployment to Iraq were assessed within a week of redeployment and again four months later and were found to have increased significantly during this interval (Bliese et al., 2007). As has been suggested with regard to PTSD, individuals may underreport depressive symptoms immediately upon return from deployment to avert adverse consequences of screening positive for depression, such as experiencing a delay in reuniting with one's family. However, it is also possible that depressive symptoms do increase during the first few months of reintegration.

Several factors may increase risk of depression among servicemembers. Combat-related deployment to Iraq or Afghanistan has been associated with increased risk of depression across military branches (Wells et al., 2010). In addition, the odds of having depression have been shown to be higher for Marine and Army personnel compared with Navy and Air Force personnel (Shen et al., 2012). Furthermore, servicemembers who are enlisted rank, female, and Hispanic/Latino have been shown to be at greater risk of probable depression (Schell and Marshall, 2008).[4]

Depression is highly comorbid, i.e., tends to co-occur, with several other psychological and physical conditions, including PTSD, substance use disorders, and chronic musculoskeletal pain. Estimates of comorbidity vary, but in the general population, 48 percent of individuals with PTSD had depression compared with 12 percent of individuals without PTSD (Kessler et al., 1995). In a military sample, approximately 65 percent of servicemembers who met criteria for probable PTSD also met criteria for probable MDD (Schell and Marshall, 2008). The high rates of co-occurrence between depression and PTSD may be partially explained by overlap in symptoms across these conditions (e.g., diminished interest, sleep problems). Similarly,

---

[4] Note that being female and of Hispanic ethnicity are documented risk factors for depression in the civilian literature (Nolen-Hoeksema, 2001; Dunlop et al., 2003).

depression and substance use disorders tend to co-occur. In the general population, individuals with substance use disorders are 14 times more likely to have MDD than individuals without substance use disorder (Grant et al., 2004). Finally, in a sample of patients with chronic musculoskeletal pain, 55.4 percent met criteria for MDD (Dersh, Gatchel, Polatin, and Mayer, 2002).

Substance Use and Abuse

Alcohol use and problems can be viewed on a continuum ranging from light to heavy alcohol use and mild to severe problems, with abuse and dependency at later ends of the continuum (IOM, 1990). Heavy alcohol use has been shown to be associated with costly outcomes. For example, among Air Force personnel, heavy drinking was associated with significant productivity loss (Mattiko et al., 2011).

Overall, the rate of heavy alcohol use and binge drinking among U.S. military personnel has increased from 1998 to 2008 (Bray et al., 2010). Several studies have examined how common drinking and binge drinking are among recently deployed servicemembers across the branches of service. For example, in a nationally representative sample of veterans and civilians, Ramchand et al. (2011) found that rates of drinking and binge drinking among previously deployed military personnel were similar to those among civilian populations, but that drinking varied significantly by branch of service. Men currently or formerly in the Air Force tended to drink less and binge drink less frequently than members in other military branches (Ramchand et al. 2011).

Several factors increase the likelihood of drinking among military personnel including younger age, being single, the number of traumas experienced, combat exposure, the number of months deployed, and co-occurring PTSD or depression (Bohnert et al, 2012; Burnett-Zeigler et al, 2011; Jacobson et al., 2008; Marshall et al, 2012; Ramchand et al., 2008). Among active-duty Air Force members, both a higher number of deployments and higher total cumulative time deployed were associated with up to a 23 percent higher likelihood of developing a postdeployment alcohol problem (Spera et al., 2011). In one study evaluating soldiers returning from combat in OIF, 62 percent of soldiers with current alcohol use disorders had the disorder before deployment, and 38 percent of soldiers developed new onset alcohol use disorders postdeployment (Kehle et al., 2012). Whether a servicemember develops alcohol use disorders following deployment may be associated with the onset of co-occurring mental health disorders (Jacobson et al., 2008). Clearly, rates of heavy alcohol use, binge drinking, and alcohol use disorders are prevalent in the military where rates of co-occurring mental health disorders and other factors interface and increase the risk of future problems.

Consequences of Comorbid PTSD and Depression

Some evidence suggests that comorbid PTSD and depression have more negative consequences than either diagnosis alone. In one study, veterans in a VA setting with comorbid depression and PTSD had more severe depression, lower social support, more suicide ideation, and more frequent primary care and mental health care visits compared with individuals with depression only (Campbell et al., 2007). Another study found that individuals with these dual diagnoses had more severe symptoms and lower levels of functioning (Shalev et al., 1998). In addition, more frequent rates of service use suggest that individuals with comorbid PTSD and depression require more treatment visits or specialized care, which may have implications for staff training and costs of treatment. These consequences are costly to individuals, their families, and society. With more complex symptoms and poorer functioning, individuals are likely to be at risk for social and occupational problems that generate further stressors.

Physical Health

Although psychological injuries are characteristic of the current conflicts (Tanielian and Jaycox, 2008; see also IOM, 2010) and known issues for our sample of airmen, some consideration of physical health issues is essential as well. General physical injuries are of concern among the combat injured, and the current conflicts have been characterized by the numbers of people who survive injuries that would have been fatal in other wars (as noted in Tanielian and Jaycox, 2008; IOM, 2010). However, we discuss specifically one type of physical injury, another "invisible wound," traumatic brain injury (TBI) (Tanielian and Jaycox, 2008).

Traumatic Brain Injury

Research indicates that between 10 and 20 percent of servicemembers returning from the Iraq and Afghanistan wars have experienced an event consistent with a TBI during deployment (Hoge, 2008; Schell and Marshall, 2008). Among servicemembers who have been wounded in Iraq or Afghanistan, TBI is the most prevalent injury (IOM, 2010). TBI results from the application of physical force or rapid acceleration/deceleration forces (e.g., mechanical trauma) that produce immediate impairment in cognitive and/or physical function, e.g., feeling dazed or confused, losing consciousness, suffering memory loss (Arciniegas et al., 2005). The majority of TBI cases (i.e., 70–80 percent) are considered to be mild (Jennett, 1996, 1998), and, of these mild cases, the vast majority (80 percent or greater) will experience resolution of TBI-related impairment within a year of the TBI (Dikmen et al., 2001). However, TBI can result in severe impairment and chronic disability (National Center for Injury Prevention and Control, 2010). TBI is also often comorbid with other mental health and substance use problems including PTSD and

MDD (see, e.g., Corrigan and Cole, 2008; Rogers and Read, 2007; Vasterling, Verfaellie, and Sullivan, 2009). Existing research suggests that the occurrence of TBI may alter the course of mental health conditions to the extent that it alters cognitive processing and emotion regulation and that they remain disrupted in the aftermath of the injury (Vasterling et al., 2009).

Other Relevant Domains of Functioning

The challenges described in preceding sections suggest that reintegration of servicemembers returning from Iraq and Afghanistan will not be easy. Mental and physical health concerns are not the only trials these servicemembers face, however. Returning veterans who are struggling with reintegration challenges such as PTSD, MDD, and TBI may face decreased quality of life. This decrement may extend far beyond the immediate issues of mental and physical health. Reintegration involves wellness on a number of interrelated fronts (Berglass and Harrell, 2012; Ramchand et al., 2008). Here, we briefly address three of them: social functioning and interpersonal relationships, employment and financial issues, and housing instability.

Social Functioning and Interpersonal Relationships

Social support has been shown to relieve the effects of various social stressors, such as unemployment or financial stress, and mitigate negative physical and mental health outcomes. We first describe how social support is defined. We then describe how research on the effect of postdeployment TBI, depression, PTSD, and reintegration stressors on veterans' relationships with friends and family members can illuminate the nature of the effects of social support on reintegration.

Social support can be defined in different ways. Generally speaking, social support is characterized by two or more individuals relating to each other (ideally, in a positive manner). This can be in the context of a marriage, a familial relationship, or in the framework of a service provider and recipient, as may be the case for programs such as AFW2 and similar wounded warrior support programs. Although not consistently a focus in this research domain, the source of support matters (Sarason and Sarason, 2006). Often, published interventions focus on support provided by strangers (Cohen, 2004) and in some cases these can actually be more effective than support provided by close relationships (i.e., marital) (Sarason and Sarason).

Two common approaches to defining social support in the literature are structural and functional (Cohen, Gottlieb, and Underwood, 2000; Cohen and Wills, 1985). As noted by Cohen and Wills in their seminal 1985 review, the structural approach focuses upon the *existence* of support relationships (i.e., marital and familial and other ties), while the functional approach considers the *functions* those relationships fulfill. They also note that measuring the bare existence of social relationships is typically a poor proxy for actually assessing the functions they provide.

The functional approach may be further subdivided into the types of functions provided by these interpersonal relationships. One is emotional support, characterized by having someone who listens to problems and provides indications of caring and compassion. Another is instrumental support, characterized by the provision of tangible resources such as financial assistance or shelter. A third is informational support, characterized by the provision of information and guidance. A fourth is other functions, such as companionship and validation (Cohen, 2004; Taylor, 2011; Wills and Shrinar, 2000). Social support interests researchers because of its documented effect on physical and mental health (e.g., Cohen, 2004; Cohen, Gottlieb, and Underwood, 2000). Cohen and Wills (1985; see also Wills and Shrinar, 2000) note that emotional support is broadly useful, but other types of support may also be relevant depending on the topic under study. For example, in a population at high risk for disability, financial concerns, and similar challenges, instrumental support may be important as well.

Social support and interpersonal relationships affect health through multiple means, including directly increasing well-being and buffering the effects of stress—that is, they enable individuals to cope with stress including traumatic events (Cohen, 2004; Cohen, Gottlieb, and Underwood, 2000; Cohen and Wills, 1985; Taylor, 2011). The presence of social ties has been linked to myriad health effects, including overall mortality (Taylor, 2011).

In a meta-analysis of a wide array of risk factors for PTSD, including sociodemographic characteristics, trauma history and severity, psychiatric history, life stress, and lack of social support, lack of social support was the most strongly related risk factor for PTSD (Brewin et al., 2000).[5] Another meta-analysis that covered a somewhat different set of risk factors also identified social support deficits as a risk factor for PTSD and found that lack of social support seemed to be a stronger predictor of PTSD with the passage of more time since the traumatic event; the authors suggest that presence of social support may serve as secondary prevention and mitigate the consequences of the trauma (Ozer et al., 2003).

Guay et al. (2006) reviewed the literature and suggested that the avenue by which social support may affect PTSD is by way of appraisal of the trauma, that is, supporters' reactions to sufferer's descriptions of the experience may affect the way sufferers process and reframe the trauma (in either a positive or negative manner). Another study found

---

[5] Studies may be prospective, in which data on risk factors were collected prior to the traumatic event, or retrospective, in which information on both risk factors and PTSD are collected after the event. Note that although the number of prospective studies was small, the effect size did not vary by prospective versus retrospective study design.

that, over time, the relationship between social support and PTSD may change such that social support may provide an initial buffer for a trauma, and, as time passes, PTSD symptoms themselves may affect social support such that they drive supporters away (Kaniasty and Norris, 2008). The exact mechanisms by which social support affects PTSD are still unclear, particularly when effects over time are considered. However, the weight of these studies suggests that social support is an important variable to consider when examining a sample with a known high rate of PTSD and potentially other psychological and physical injuries.

Insufficient social support and interaction may also be key in the development and maintenance of depression (Lara and Klein, 1999; Star and Davila, 2008). In addition, one study on veteran homelessness post-Vietnam found that the greatest risk factors for homelessness were related to social isolation (lack of social support and being unmarried after the first years of discharge) (Rosenheck and Fontana, 1994). These findings in concert with the information on PTSD and social support suggest that the role of social support in reintegration warrants additional consideration. Moreover, as noted above, programmatic provision of social support is often studied: that is, social support by service providers such as those in the reintegration programs provided to airmen by the Air Force.

Unemployment and Financial Issues

Work provides many benefits, is often central to how adults view themselves, and hence is a relevant reintegration domain area. As outlined by Hulin (2002; see also Arvey et al., 2004; Fouad and Bynner, 2008; Warr, 1987), it provides identity, structure to time, a source of relationships, and a pecuniary benefit. It is a noted factor in transition to adulthood (e.g., Shanahan, 2000). For those with mental illness, employment may be seen as aiding recovery (Dunn et al. 2008), facilitating reintegration into society, and having many other benefits (Corbiere and LeComte, 2009). Unemployment describes the situation of individuals who lose their job and possibly their work identity. Research does not typically define this term further, but unplanned job loss is most often seen as stressful and is an issue with continuing currency in the present economic climate (Wanberg, 2012). As noted by Nichols, Mitchell, and Lindner (2013), past studies of unemployment suggest that layoffs for cause, perhaps including unfitting-for-work conditions as in our sample of airmen with combat-related injuries, may have greater negative sequelae than layoffs for external factors such as factory closings.

What role does unemployment play in the context of this analysis, given that our research effort is focused on individuals who are employed at the time of their injury? If a servicemember's condition renders him or her unable to perform military duty, he or she may be considered for retirement or separation (Department of Defense Directive [DoDD] 1332.18). According to AFI 41-210, "[servicemembers] identified with a potential Service-disqualifying medical diagnosis, condition, physical or mental limitation will be evaluated, and when indicated, referred through the Disability Evaluation System (DES)" (p. 173). Relevant here is the fact that some mental health disorders (including both PTSD and MDD) make airmen eligible for this determination of unfitness:

> Individuals who experience recurrent depression or anxiety disorders, require psychiatric medication for greater than one year, who have been hospitalized for a psychiatric condition. …These cases warrant careful consideration of fitness for duty, worldwide assignability and deployability, given that adequate mental health support may not be available in all locations (AFI 48-123, p. 46).

Thus, one concern for veterans with PTSD, MDD, TBI, and other potentially disabling injuries is loss of military employment and the necessity of gaining new employment when disabled, in addition to concern about the disability itself.

More generally, employment and financial well-being of veterans are a concern because PTSD has a documented relationship with poor employment outcomes, based on research done with Vietnam veterans (see, e.g., Savoca and Rosenheck, 2000; Smith, Schnurr, and Rosenheck, 2005). Cook's (2006) review of employment barriers among those with mental illness suggests that presence of *any* mental health condition was likely to be related to a lower likelihood of employment (different surveys summarized had estimates of 48 to 73 percent employment for those with mental health difficulties, whereas those surveys' estimates for employment for well workers ranged between 76 and 87 percent).

Moreover, presence of any mental health condition was associated with lower income for those who were employed (Cook, 2006; see also Banerjee, Chatterji, and Lahiri, 2013). People with various mental health conditions may also be less productive at work (see, e.g., Adler et al., 2008; Cook, 2006; Ettner, Frank, and Kessler, 1997; Schultz and Edington, 2007). Indeed, Banerjee et al. indicate that more effective mental illness treatment would reduce the societal costs of absenteeism by $18.9 billion in 2002 dollars. Finally, Cook reports that those with mental illness represent the largest group of public income support beneficiaries among those of working age.

Notwithstanding these statistics, Cook's review indicates that many of those with mental health conditions want to work. Moreover, Bond, Resnick, et al. (2001) found that competitive employment improved a number of outcomes for participants with a variety of psychiatric disorders. Commonly cited barriers to gaining employment among this population are lower educational attainment, lower productivity, labor market dynamics, and failure to receive effective vocational or clinical services (see, e.g., Cook, 2006). Discrimination and stigma are also factors (see, e.g., Colella and Bruyere, 2011).[6]

A substantial literature exists on the consequences of unemployment, which include detriments to both psychological and physical well-being (McKee-Ryan et al., 2005). McKee-Ryan et al. analytically summarized this literature, focusing on indices of psychological well-being, which included the Beck Depression Inventory and the General Health Questionnaire, among other screeners for depression and anxiety. Mental health during unemployment was positively and significantly related to other variables including social support and financial resources, and negatively and significantly related to perceived centrality of work to life and the length of unemployment. McKee-Ryan et al. also found that the relationship between unemployment and mental health did not vary depending on generosity of unemployment benefits (though there may have been some restriction of range in this analysis, which would have limited their ability to detect such variation). Wanberg's more recent 2012 summary of the unemployment literature notes that unemployment has also been associated with negative outcomes such as suicide and decrements in physical health (c.f. Nichols, Mitchell, and Lindner 2013). Nichols et al. considered the long-term unemployed (defined as those unemployed six months or more), and noted its association with decrements in well-being, income, and work skills. These decrements include lower incomes upon finally gaining employment that may be quite persistent.[7] With regard to the specific experiences of servicemembers, as noted by Heaton et al. (2012), injuries incurred during deployment have broad effects on traditional economic indicators such as financial well-being and employment. Specifically, for those categorized as having more serious injuries, they documented a substantial loss in income. This loss in income was primarily because of separation or retirement from military service as a consequence of the injury. They note that at least in the initial years of study, on average, disability income compensated, or more than compensated, for these losses in household income. However, they speculate that over time, given removal from the workforce and the wage increases customarily experienced

---

[6] In the domain of civilian legislation, protection from discrimination is available under various laws, including the Americans with Disabilities Act (Colella and Bruyere, 2011; Paludi et al., 2011). Note that for the military context, to the extent that deployment is considered an essential job function, such legislation would not apply (Gutman et al., 2011). However, in their reviews of the disability literature, multiple authors have noted the substantive difficulties faced in gaining and maintaining employment when disabled despite these legislative remedies (Colella and Bruyere, 2001; Cook, 2006; Paludi et al., 2011). These authors also note that issues of discrimination are particularly pertinent for disabilities based on mental illness, which are more stigmatized than physical disabilities.

[7] They also note that there may not be a direct causal connection between long-term unemployment and subsequent negative outcomes but that both the unemployment and the outcomes might be caused by a third factor. They note that the literature disentangling the direct effects of unemployment lengths from other potential causal factors is not comprehensive.

while in the workforce, disability incomes would fall behind the lifetime income ordinarily expected.

Although the population in our study represents many whose challenges are identified while they are still in service, it is worth noting that disabilities such as PTSD may not manifest before servicemembers leave service but rather months or years later. Other research is therefore relevant: Christensen and colleagues (2007) compared the earnings of those rated by the VA as service disabled (who may receive such a rating long after leaving military employ) with a comparable peer group. Those with disabilities had, on average, lower employment rates and rates of earned income, with variations for age at entry into the system, magnitude of disability rating, and body system of injury. They found that in general VA compensation enabled those with service disabilities to reach parity over lifetime earnings with those peers who did not have service-related disabilities, with exceptions. If a veteran enters the system at an earlier age, parity is not reached for those who have 100 percent disability or who are deemed to meet IU status.[8] Further, for those with a mental disability (PTSD or mental, other than PTSD), compensation falls below what would normally be expected for those who enter prior to what may be considered typical retirement years (i.e., 65+) or for those who have lower disability ratings. Although research has yet to ascertain the long-term effects of deployment-related injuries incurred in the OIF/OEF conflicts, there is evidence to support the effect of military service as a net positive over the life course on financial well-being for the general population of servicemembers (Kleykamp, 2013a and 2013b; Loughran, 2002). However, Loughran's (2002) findings indicate that the civilian earnings of military retirees are not comparable to those of their civilian peers, with greater disparities observed for more recent cohorts.

Also noted by Heaton et al. (2012), the majority of the income sources they examined, including DoD and VA disability benefits, do not penalize disabled individuals for attempting to secure civilian employment subsequent to separation and hence alleviate some concern that receipt of benefits may discourage recipients from continuing to engage in the workforce. Given the indications that employment may be beneficial for individuals with mental disability (Cook, 2006; Corbiere and LeComte, 2009), this is positive. However, as noted by McKee-Ryan et al. (2005), the search for employment can itself be demoralizing, which is only likely to be exacerbated by the presence of potentially stigmatizing disorders.

Of particular importance to psychological well-being and employment is perceived financial strain, or the extent to which individuals consider themselves to be experiencing

---

[8] IU, or individual unemployability, is a status that requires meeting certain disability criteria and being unable to engage in substantial gainful employment; it results in compensation at the 100 percent disability level.

financial difficulties. This is assessed without regard to objective indicators of financial strain. McKee-Ryan et al. (2005) noted that perceived financial strain was negatively associated with psychological well-being during unemployment. Indeed, in another meta-analysis, Kanfer, Wanberg, and Kantrowitz (2001) found that perceived financial strain was associated with greater job search behavior and shorter unemployment duration.

Housing Instability

As U.S. servicemembers return from the conflicts in Iraq and Afghanistan and leave active duty, a concern is the domain of housing instability. Homelessness has been a persistent concern within the veteran community, with veterans consistently overrepresented among homeless Americans (Perl, 2011). Increasing numbers of veterans with deployment-related risk factors (i.e., disabilities), a sluggish economy, and reduced budgets may collectively elevate the risk of homelessness among returning veterans. Thus, we examine housing stability and instability within the current context.

Defining Homelessness

Financial and other vulnerabilities may place people at risk for other negative sequelae, including housing instability (Koegel, 2004). However, defining "homeless" poses a challenge. The term "homeless" typically describes anyone without permanent housing. For example, both a person living under a bridge and a person staying in a hotel for an extended period because of a lack of permanent housing could be considered homeless under this broad definition. This ambiguity causes problems when measuring the concept of homelessness, and researchers employ a variety of more specific definitions to mitigate such problems. For example, when studying outcomes among homeless veterans using the U.S. Department of Housing and Urban Development-Veterans Affairs Supported Housing (HUD-VASH), O'Connell, Kasprow, and Rosenheck (2008) examined only those who had lived on the street or in a shelter for at least 30 days because this was a requirement of HUD-VASH (O'Connell, Kasprow, and Rosenheck, 2008). Conversely, Rosenheck and Fontana (1994) researched those who "had no regular place to live for at least a month or so." Still others define homelessness as "spending at least one night on the street, or in a shelter, mission, vehicle, public or abandoned building, or voucher hotel because they did not have a home of their own or of a family member or friend to stay in" (Kennedy et al., 2012). Clearly, these definitions can refer to people with varied housing situations, but all reflect housing instability.

To further clarify this definitional ambiguity, researchers have suggested that homelessness can be broken down into three categories defined by the amount of time one is without permanent housing. "Transitionally" homeless people have been in a situation without regular housing once for a short period before returning to permanent housing. This may include stays at a homeless shelter or in a car or hotel. "Episodically" homeless people transition in and out of homelessness with some regularity but do not stay homeless for an extended amount of time. Finally, "chronically" homeless people have been without permanent housing for at least one year or have been homeless at least four times in the past three years (Kuhn and Culhane, 1998; Perl, 2011). The researchers who derived this typology noted that, in their study, the majority of shelter resources were consumed by the chronically homeless (Kuhn and Culhane, 1998). This typology has been found useful (Leginski, 2007) although not always replicable (Burt et al., 2001).

Policymakers also wrestle with this issue when determining who should or should not receive government assistance, in some cases aiming intervention at those chronically homeless (Leginski, 2007). Various congressional actions in the past few decades have sought to provide aid to both veteran and nonveteran homeless people. The definitions contained in these laws help provide clarity to the policy-centric definition of homelessness. For example, the McKinney-Vento Homeless Assistance Act defines a homeless individual as one who lacks a fixed, regular, and adequate nighttime residence and whose nighttime residence is one of the following:

- a supervised publically or privately operated shelter designed to provide temporary living accommodations
- an institution that provides a temporary residence for individuals intended to be institutionalized
- a public or private place not designed for, nor ordinarily used as, a regular sleeping accommodation for human beings (Perl, 2011).

As noted by Burt and colleagues (2001), narrow definitions may have the drawback of focusing efforts on ameliorative rather than preventive approaches to housing instability. Other definitions do appear in different pieces of legislation that echo the common theme of housing instability. Some further acknowledge the role of substance abuse and mental health issues in homelessness (Perl, 2011). Current modifications to the original legislation expand the definition to elaborate on what locations are not normally considered regular sleeping accommodations and include government and charitably funded hotels and motels as temporary living arrangements. These modifications also include individuals in imminent danger of losing housing within two weeks (see Perl et al., 2012), and overall move the somewhat restrictive original definition toward a more inclusive one. Defining homelessness is a complex issue, and consideration of the ultimate goal of research and policy should inform approach and breadth.

Veteran homelessness has been tracked by two government entities: the VA and the Department of Housing and Urban Development (HUD). Over the years, these organizations have changed their methodologies for tracking the number of homeless veterans, leading to varying estimates. However, both agree that veteran homelessness is declining. In 2009, the VA estimated that 106,558 homeless veterans resided in the United States, down from 131,230 in 2008 (Perl, 2011). As noted by Perl, though declining in numbers, veterans are still overrepresented in the homeless population. In a more recent study, HUD found that 11.1 percent of homeless adults were veterans, although veterans constitute only 9.7 percent of the U.S. adult population. Additional studies have found that, depending on their era of service and gender, veterans can be up to three times more likely to end up homeless compared with nonveterans (Perl, 2011).

Research Findings

A considerable amount of research has been conducted to identify the factors that place veterans at increased risk for homelessness. Two general and not mutually exclusive perspectives attribute the causes either to situational or individual issues (Burt et al., 2001; Koegel, 2004). The situational, or structural, context of homelessness is defined by influences outside of the individual that contribute to a lack of permanent housing such as a slow economy, a decrease in affordable housing, and policy changes that reduced the amount of government aid available to those in poverty (Koegel, 2004). These issues take place in the world around an individual and can contribute to homelessness, especially in conjunction with problems someone might be experiencing on a personal level.

The individual issues most common among homeless veterans stem both from military service and life before the military and help create a picture of general vulnerability and risk. Research has shown that a history of trauma before joining the military, including physical or sexual abuse, life in foster care, or witnessing someone's death, is significantly related to veteran homelessness (Rosenheck and Fontana, 1994). Problems in one's life after military service that contribute to homelessness in the veteran community often include substance abuse and psychiatric disorders (Rosenheck and Fontana, 1994). A lack of steady employment has also been consistently observed in homeless veterans seeking government assistance (Perl, 2011). However, the strongest individual factor affecting veteran homelessness seems to be a lack of social support. Veterans without strong connections to friends, family, or an intimate partner are often found to have the highest risk for homelessness (Rosenheck and Fontana, 1994).

Opportunities for Intervention

Throughout this review we have considered definitions of potential risk factors or vulnerabilities. However, the knowledge that something is a risk factor makes that issue into a risk that may be mitigated: a gateway for opportunity. Thus the interrelated risk factors discussed here may function as interrelated avenues for intervention in pursuit of wellness. Taking the holistic perspective reveals that none of these areas should be viewed in isolation when considering the possibilities for intervention to improve reintegration. Failure to consider the full breadth of issues can be problematic not only in terms of realistically predicting trajectories and the levers to change those trajectories, but also in terms of considering the variety of policy levers available. Given the theoretical rationale or empirical evidence, and the interrelatedness of the factors discussed, omission of a given factor is likely to provide policy decisionmakers with a potentially flawed picture of what interventions may be best, and why. To present an accurate perspective to guide interventions, it is important to include a breadth of domains for consideration wherever possible. Moreover, all of these domains may be considered to be indicators of resilience as well as risk. To the extent that the AFW2 and AFRCC programs, among others, seek to assist in a beneficial reintegration process, improvement in any of these domains could represent a positive programmatic outcome.

A holistic perspective is warranted for the current project even though some of the factors under consideration may not have a strong evidence base to inform policy recommendations. Traditional services for the combat injured may not always include efforts in a given domain. However, the literature described above indicates that all may be relevant, and we have included them for consideration here, and in our baseline survey effort; as noted, they not only indicate risk, but also are relevant to programmatic outcomes. Evidence-based treatments (EBTs), i.e., treatments whose efficacy has been demonstrated in well-designed research studies, are available to alleviate some of the challenges faced in the domains of different variable sets. The evidence base is particularly strong in the realm of mental health, where a push toward interventions with demonstrable efficacy has been under way for some time.

Mental and Physical Health

EBTs are available for PTSD (Bradley et al., 2005; IOM, 2012). The VA and DoD in particular have institutionalized evidence-based care for PTSD through a shared set of guidelines on PTSD management, VA/DoD Clinical Practice Guideline for the Management of Post-Traumatic Stress (The Management of Post-Traumatic Stress Working Group, 2010). The VA/DoD guidelines for management of PTSD recommend trauma-focused psychotherapies such as prolonged exposure (PE), cognitive processing therapy (CPT), and eye movement desensitization and reprocessing (EMDR) and stress inoculation. Psychotropic medications such as selective serotonin reuptake inhibitors (SSRIs) are also recommended.

Similarly, EBTs are available for other mental and physical health issues. With regard to MDD, they are institutionalized in the VA/DoD Clinical Practice Guideline for the Management of Major Depressive Disorder (The Management of MDD Working Group, 2009). The VA/DoD guidelines recommend psychotropic medications such as SSRIs and serotonin norepinephrine reuptake inhibitors (SNRIs), as well as cognitive behavioral therapy (CBT) and interpersonal therapy (IPT), which have been shown to be efficacious (e.g., Anderson, 2000; Butler et al., 2006; Feijo de Mello et al., 2005). EBTs are also available for substance use and are outlined in the VA/DoD guidelines for clinical care (VA/DoD Clinical Practice Guideline for Management of Substance Use Disorders, 2009). EBTs for substance use include pharmacotherapy such as opiate agonist therapy (OAT) and psychosocial interventions such as cognitive behavioral coping skills training. These treatments are supported in the literature (Farre et al., 2002; Fischer, 2006; Johnson et al., 2000; Ball et al., 2007; Carroll et al., 2006; Wilbourne, 2005). For mild TBI, suggestions include methods to cope with the consequences of TBI and promote the recovery process such as early education about the injury and pharmacological or behavioral therapy as needed to treat the various symptoms of TBI (VA/DoD Clinical Practice Guideline for Management of Concussion/Mild Traumatic Brain Injury, 2009). While the evidence base for these suggestions does not yet support meta-analyses, individual studies demonstrating the benefits of education are available (Wade, Crawford, et al., 1997; Paniak, Toller-Lobe, et al., 1998; Wade, King, et al., 1998; Paniak, Toller-Lobe, et al., 2000; Ponsford, Willmott, et al., 2002; Warden, 2006). Additionally, in limited studies, cognitive behavioral therapy has been shown to be effective to aid TBI patients with ailments like insomnia (Ouellet and Moria, 2007). Pharmacotherapy has further been shown effective in the treatment of various consequences of TBI including aggression and information processing (Warden et al., 2006).

The VA and DoD formally advocate evidence-based care. However, the extent to which providers in these systems are consistently practicing EBTs and implementing EBTs with fidelity to the treatment protocol (i.e., the way the treatment was designed to be delivered) is unknown. This uncertainty is because of the lack of systematic tracking of the quality of mental health care provided within the VA and DoD (IOM, 2012). On the civilian side, indications that evidence-based care and treatment are being translated from the research base to community practice are even less promising (President's New Freedom Commission on Mental Health, 2003).

Moreover, although evidence-based treatments exist, several barriers may prevent servicemembers or veterans with mental health concerns from obtaining high-quality care (IOM, 2012; Tanielian and Jaycox, 2008). For instance, shortages of qualified mental health treatment providers in some geographic areas of the United States limit access to care (Burnam et al., 2008). In studies of previously deployed OEF/OIF servicemembers and veterans, institutional and cultural concerns about the adverse effects of receiving mental health treatment on one's career and coworkers' perceptions have been consistently reported (Hoge et al., 2004; Schell and Marshall, 2008; Vaughan et al., 2011; Vogt, 2011). Other commonly endorsed concerns include concerns about the side effects of medication (Schell and Marshall, 2008; Vaughan et al., 2011), personal beliefs about mental health and mental health care (Vogt, 2011), and difficulty scheduling an appointment (Hoge et al., 2004). Little is known about the barriers to mental health treatment encountered by severely wounded veterans, and documentation of the types and prevalence of barriers encountered by this population is needed (IOM, 2012).

The evidence base for some other areas is less thoroughly explored than in the domains of mental and physical health, although quite often many programs are available in other domains to address needs. Although the medical and mental health literature are replete with randomized control trials comparing two modes of treatment, and an accumulation of evidence allows for meta-analyses of effects over multiple studies, other relevant fields are still in the process of accumulating quality evidence for effectiveness. We now describe research on reintegration challenges encountered in nonmedical domains, specifically social functioning, employment, finances, and housing instability.

Social Functioning and Interpersonal Relationships

Multiple interventions exist that attempt to improve emotional social support. Hogan et al. (2002) summarized the literature and found significant heterogeneity in successful health outcomes among people involved in a similarly wide variety of group interventions. These include friends and family in behavioral training, self-help groups, organized support from psychiatrists, psychologists, etc., or support skills training programs with certified professionals that follow a defined curriculum, individual-level interventions (including friends or family in one-on-one discussion with professionals, peer groups, or one-on-one support skills training programs), and combination therapy that involves both group- and individual-level intervention. Given the heterogeneity of interventions found in their overview, Hogan et al. were not able to categorize specific practices as evidence based, but they were able to suggest that some type of social support intervention shows promise in a general sense. Supportive interpersonal relationships include service provider and recipient, as may be the case for the involvement programs such as AFW2. In some cases support from providers may be more effective than support from close relationships (Sarason and Sarason, 2006). More directly relevant to our sample of combat-injured airmen, incorporation of the social support network into therapy itself has also been suggested for veterans with PTSD (e.g., Sherman, Zanotti, and Jones, 2005).

Unemployment and Financial Issues

Employment interventions are also available, and the evidence base for these interventions is the strongest we examined aside from that for various mental health interventions. In general, employment interventions are based in one of two literatures: the broader literature on unemployment or the psychiatric treatment/vocational rehabilitation literature. As summarized by Wanberg (2012), the broader literature on unemployment suggests that interventions to bolster self-efficacy may be tenable and, indeed, some have been developed. One program of study has collected an evidence base to support a particular intervention (the University of Michigan JOBS program) aimed at enabling the unemployed to find jobs by identifying marketable skills, learning how to locate job opportunities, identifying methods of self-presentation, and becoming inoculated against the demoralizing nature of the job search itself (Price, Vinokur, and Friedland, 2002). There is some evidence that those participants who subsequently became employed worked more and had fewer changes of employer (Vinokur et al., 1991), and a follow-up study indicated that those with the greatest risk of depressive symptoms were most likely to benefit from the program (Vinokur, Price, and Schul, 1995). Wanberg (2012) noted other potential intervention avenues, including research that suggested that self-presentation tactics lead to interview success (and might be targets for training), as well as other research documenting interventions to improve self-efficacy in the job search and goal-oriented behavior such as documentation of job search activities.

Evidence from the psychiatric intervention/vocational rehabilitation literature largely supports a model of supported employment. The model is characterized by consideration of individual job seeker interests and abilities in the job search process, preference for competitive community employment as opposed to employment in more sheltered programs, rapid job search to alleviate waning job seeker interest in job acquisition, integration of mental health and employment intervention efforts, and continued support once employment is attained (Bond, 2004). Bond also summarized evidence in support of these principles, characterizing the support as ranging from strong (for rapid job search) to weak (for time-unlimited support). More recently, Cook et al. (2006) indicated that participants enrolled in variations of supported employment programs fared better than did control subjects when accounting for the local unemployment rate. Resnick, Rosenheck, and Drebing (2006) indicated that the key ingredients of successful programs included competitive community employment and aggressive outreach to veterans.

Housing Instability

Many avenues also exist to help veterans struggling with homelessness. The VA and HUD have the most involvement with improving the housing situation of homeless veterans. The VA has many programs to help homeless veterans obtain health care, find stable housing, gain employment, and get off the streets. In fact, the VA stated in 2009 that it aimed to end veteran homelessness within five years (Perl, 2011). Some of these programs include Health Care for Homeless Veterans, Domiciliary Care for Homeless Veterans, and the Compensated Work Therapy Program, among others (Perl, 2011). One program that has shown particular promise in housing homeless veterans is the aforementioned HUD-VASH. In this collaboration between the VA and HUD, veterans can receive vouchers for subsidized housing along with counseling and other services that will improve their chances of obtaining stable housing. Research has shown that veterans enrolled in HUD-VASH are more likely to stay continuously housed longer (O'Connell et al., 2008) and are less likely to experience substance abuse (Perl, 2011).

Summary

Einstein is credited with saying that "Everything should be as simple as possible, but no simpler." This observation applies naturally to an examination of processes such as reintegration. However, reintegration is by its nature complicated, and a holistic model of reintegration therefore is required to examine the process appropriately.

Hence, we have delineated the domains that should affect the process and describe some of the evidence for their inclusion. Mental health is a key issue for servicemember reintegration in general and for our sample of Air Force wounded warriors in particular because of the high prevalence of this injury in the sample, and it can have a cascading effect on several other types of outcomes. As discussed, conditions may co-occur, and a given illness such as PTSD should not be considered in isolation. Physical health and wounds of war are also relevant and affect well-being. Other issues that merit consideration based on the literature include social functioning and interpersonal relationships, employment and financial issues, and housing instability. Although rigorous longitudinal research on these topics is relatively scarce, the evidence available suggests that these domains will affect each other over time and that relationships are likely to be complex. Moreover, to the extent that all are factors in a robust reintegration process, all provide outcome information regarding the success of programs such as AFW2, AFRCC, and the VA's programs. Some of these domains have a robust evidence base that supports specific intervention, while others are still accumulating such evidence. However, even when a strong evidence base exists, as it does for mental health, in some cases having specific interventions and recommended courses of action is not enough. Therefore barriers to care warrant exploration as well to understand the process.

This literature review informs our general approach to the analysis by establishing the case for examining a holistic suite of relevant domains. Moreover, the relevance of particular domains in the literature specifically influenced the variables we included in our survey of wounded warriors, both by helping us determine which domains were pertinent to include and how we measured these domains in our survey. Perspective on the holistic reintegration process as it is understood through the literature in turn affects the conclusions we can draw based on the included domains. Finally, to the extent that an evidence base for intervention exists for these domains, that evidence base undergirds our implementation recommendations. Although we included measures of the majority of the above variables in our survey, we present only the most essential risk factors and directly actionable findings in the main text of the results. The remainder of survey results is presented in Appendix C. Although the results from the present survey represent a baseline snapshot, given that the domains of investigation are relevant indicators of both risk and resilience, improvement in the domains of study suggest that the reintegration of the airmen in our population is going more smoothly, while a decrement may indicate that a stronger policy intervention is warranted.

3. Survey Method

This chapter provides an overview of our survey procedure and content. The previous chapter includes a general discussion of relevant domains, and we provide more details on the specifics of measurement here. The chapter begins with a description of the survey participants. Second, it recounts how we administered the survey. The third section summarizes the measures we employed for the outcomes or areas of interest as suggested by our literature review and holistic approach to reintegration.

Sampling of Participants

As the Air Force's focus was on airmen injured in combat, we pursued airmen enrolled in one of the programs developed to assist them, the AFW2 program. This focus was optimal in the sense that all in the frame were eligible (i.e., all had been determined to have combat- or hostile-related injuries), and relatively up-to-date contact information was available for all participants. This information was particularly important in the case of retirees whose records are typically not current in the personnel data system.

The AFW2 program, stood up in 2005 as Palace HART (Helping Airmen Recover Together), was renamed in 2007 as the Air Force Wounded Warrior program. Throughout, however, the intent remained constant: to assist airmen in transition and reintegration after their injury or illness. At the time the survey was fielded, the eligibility requirements were described as follows:

> An Airman who has a combat/hostile-related injury or illness requiring long-term care that may require a MEB/PEB [Medical Evaluation Board/Physical Evaluation Board] to determine fitness for duty. This includes: A combat/hostile-related injury resulting from hazardous service or performance of duty under conditions simulating war or through an instrumentality of war. (AFW2 website, undated.)

There is no minimum disability rating for eligibility, and enrollment could occur through several channels, including self-referral, casualty list seriously injured (SI) and very seriously injured (VSI) status;[1] referral from command or medical community; and referral from the Disability Evaluation System. When a name enters the AFW2 system from one of the referral sources, available records systems (including casualty and deployment records, the DES, and other personnel records) are accessed, and the

---

[1] SI is "classified by medical authorities to be of such severity that there is cause for immediate concern, but there is no imminent danger to life"; and VSI is "classified by medical authorities to be of such severity that life is imminently endangered" (Joint Publication 1-02).

information is integrated to form an initial intake packet. This information is supplemented by a telephone intake interview. According to program personnel, a better-safe-than-sorry approach is adopted in terms of determination of combat- or hostile-relatedness of injury. In some cases, this determination is not confirmed, and a judgment is made that the airman is not eligible for AFW2 services. However, we were told that this is a rare occurrence.

As no minimum disability rating is required to obtain services from AFW2, its population of benefit recipients includes separatees. These individuals have a disability rating of less than 30 percent and receive a lump sum payment (the amount is determined by a formula and considers the disability rating and the servicemember's tenure and base pay) upon separation. As these separatees are not receiving substantial ongoing pecuniary benefits, they are considered members of the general population rather than current servicemembers or "actual" benefit recipients and were excluded from our sample.[2]

Thus, the sample for our project consisted of the 872 enrollees of the Air Force Wounded Warrior Program who were either medically retired or in the process of undergoing evaluation for medical retirement due to combat or related injuries and illness. The majority of individuals (71 percent) had primary injuries of a psychological rather than a physical (29 percent) nature. For most, the concern that brought them into the program was PTSD. Given the relatively small number of potential participants, we chose to take a census rather than to select a subsample from the frame. Of the 872 airmen who were invited to participate, 493 accepted.

Procedure for Administering the Survey

Initial invitations were mailed to potential participants' home addresses. These invitations included instructions on how to complete the survey by web, if desired, through a unique survey login code. Throughout the invitation and consent procedures, participants were assured that their information would be seen by the Air Force only in the aggregate, that participation would not affect their benefits, and that a Certificate of Confidentiality from the U.S. Department of Health and Human Services and memoranda of understanding (MOUs) with Air Force sponsor offices had been obtained to ensure confidentiality. These assurances were intended to alleviate some of the known concerns regarding stigmatization of mental health problems both in the military and in the larger population as well as to inform participants that their participation or lack thereof would not have an adverse effect. Ultimately, that assurance to participants is one of the

---

[2] Note that it is still possible that these separatees may later be given a rating for the sum total of their service-connected conditions from the VA that is a higher rating than that provided by the Air Force at time of separation, which assesses only unfitting conditions.

strongest protections for our results in that it reduces motivation to attempt to skew results in either direction: either to minimize or emphasize symptoms and other challenges being faced in participants' daily lives.

Approximately one week following the initial distribution of recruitment materials, potential participants were contacted by phone and invited to complete the survey by phone. During that contact, participants were able to indicate that they had already started the web survey or were planning to do so. Those who preferred to participate by phone were able to participate then or schedule a call-back if the initial call was made at an inconvenient time. In circumstances where individuals were not interested in participating by phone, they were given information on how to participate over the web.

Survey items were worded identically across the web and telephone survey administration modes. However, instructions were modified as needed to accommodate differences in aural versus visual presentation of survey items, e.g., for the measure of PTSD symptoms, instructions read by interviewers administering the phone survey began, "Now I am going to read you a list of reactions that airmen sometimes experience following deployment or in response to other stressful life experiences…," whereas instructions given to web survey respondents began "The following is a list of reactions…" The survey took approximately 45 minutes to complete in either mode.

The survey was in the field from September 2 through October 31, 2011, and as noted, during that period, 493 airmen accessed the survey. Due to skip patterns within the survey designed to minimize respondent burden, not all participants saw all items. For example, participants who had not received AFW2 services were not asked about satisfaction with such services. If a participant indicated that he or she was not employed, he or she was not asked about work presenteeism, performance, job satisfaction, or the like. If employed, he or she was not asked about perceived barriers to employment. Approximately 120 items were seen by all participants. More specifics on amount and treatment of missing data are provided in the next chapter.

Measures Used in the Survey

We used well-validated measures of the constructs of interest when such measures were available. When well-validated measures were not available, e.g., to assess utilization and perceptions of the Air Force Wounded Warrior and Air Force Recovery Care Coordinator programs, we created items to tap the construct of interest. Our points of contact in the AFW2 and AFRCC programs and the Air Force Directorate of Services (AF/A1S) reviewed early drafts of the survey and provided feedback on the overall approach and specific sections and items, which was incorporated into the final version. We also employed limited cognitive interviewing with a few survey research experts at RAND to hone the survey. Table 3.1 summarizes the measures and their provenances.

Detailed descriptions of the measures' psychometric properties and scoring instructions for variables derived from the measures are contained in Appendix A. The final survey is contained in Appendix B. We also examined mode effects for the measures used in the survey. After performing a Bonferroni correction to adjust the significance level for the number of tests performed (85), we found that those who answered on the web were more likely to indicate that an advocate would be helpful; that there was a point in the past year where they desired but did not receive assistance; and that they indicated higher work involvement. As, in general, there were relatively few distinctions between mode, and we wanted to maximize our power to detect theoretically meaningful effects, we combined participants in subsequent sections.

Table 3.1. Survey Measures Overview

Outcome/Area	Description	Measure and Supporting Citations
Air Force service history	AF component, time since separation or retirement, etc.	Some items created for this project, some adapted from Invisible Wounds survey (Schell and Marshall, 2008)
Trauma history	History of traumatic stressors (Criterion A of PTSD diagnosis)	Created for this project based on an item used in the Invisible Wounds study (Tanielian and Jaycox, 2008)
Post traumatic symptom severity	Extent to which respondent has been bothered by symptoms of PTSD during the past month. There are three primary groups of PTSD symptoms: intrusive thoughts, memories, and recollections of the traumatic event; avoidance of things that remind the respondent of the traumatic event; and emotional and/or physiological arousal when reminded of the event	PTSD Checklist (PCL; Weathers et al., 1993)
Depressive symptoms	Extent to which respondent has been bothered by symptoms of depression during the past two weeks	Patient Health Questionnaire-8 (PHQ-8; Spitzer et al., 1999)
Alcohol use	Frequency of alcohol consumption and problems related to alcohol use during the past six months	Alcohol Use Disorder Identification Test-Alcohol Consumption (AUDIT-C; Bush et al., 1998)
Drug use	Use of drugs other than alcohol and problems related to drug use during the past six months	Adapted from Needs Assessment of New York State Veterans (Vaughan et al., 2011)

Outcome/Area	Description	Measure and Supporting Citations
Potential traumatic brain injury	Whether respondent experienced an event indicative of potential traumatic brain injury, as indicated by being dazed and confused, not remembering the injury, or experiencing a loss of consciousness following an injury sustained during deployment	Brief Traumatic Brain Injury Scale (BTBIS); Schwab et al., 2007)
General health	Perception of overall health	SF-36; Ware et al., 1993
Role limitations due to physical health	Extent to which respondent is physically limited in his/her ability to perform different activities	SF-36; Ware et al., 1993
Mental health treatment history, barriers, and preferences	Mental health services received, barriers to obtaining mental health treatment, type and setting of treatment desired if respondent wanted treatment	Created for this project, some adapted from Invisible Wounds (Schell and Marshall, 2008)
Basic information about marital status and family	Marital status, number of dependents, family members living in the same household, family member that most often helps airman deal with problems, etc.	Created for this project with assistance from program personnel
Relationship satisfaction	Degree of satisfaction with relationship with significant other or primary supporter (if respondent does not have a significant other)	Johnson, D. R., 1995
Social support	Extent to which respondent perceives that different types of social support are available from people in his/her life	Reliable Alliance and Attachment subscales of the Social Provisions Scale (SPS; Cutrona and Russell, 1985)
Employment status	Whether respondent is currently working or not and how often	Needs Assessment of New York State Veterans (Vaughan et al., 2011) Invisible Wounds survey (Schell and Marshall, 2008)
Presenteeism/ absenteeism	Productivity at work, number of days missed	World Health Organization Health and Work Performance Questionnaire (WHO HPQ; Kessler et al., 2003)
Employability—work identity	Perceived importance of work/psychological investment in work	Warr et al., 1979
Job satisfaction	Degree of satisfaction with job in general	Scarpello and Campbell, 1983; Weiss et al., 1967
Barriers to employment	[If respondent is "Unemployed and looking for work" or "Disabled and not working"] Things that make it difficult for respondent to obtain employment	Adapted from the Wounded Warriors project survey (Franklin et al., 2010)
Vocational rehabilitation services utilization	Whether or not respondent has used vocational rehabilitation services	2007 President's Commission on Care for America's Returning Wounded Warriors
Income and disability compensation	Information about total household income	Invisible Wounds survey (Schell and Marshall, 2008)
Financial strain	Difficulty meeting one's financial obligations	Financial strain measure; Vinokur and Caplan (1987)

33

Outcome/Area	Description	Measure and Supporting Citations
Housing situation	Current living situation (homeless/at-risk of becoming homeless/not homeless)	Wenzel, 2005; 2010 studies
Evaluation of Air Force Wounded Warrior program	Airman's contact with AFW2; help and services the airman has received from AFW2; perceptions of AFW2's effectiveness and helpfulness and overall satisfaction with AFW2; barriers to using AFW2	Created for this project with assistance from program personnel
Evaluation of Air Force Recovery Care Coordinator program	Airman's contact with RCC program; help and services received; perceptions of program effectiveness, helpfulness; overall satisfaction with program	Created for this project with assistance from program personnel
Services and benefits received from other programs, services and benefits most desired	Services and benefits received from VA; area in which respondent would most like assistance (whether already receiving or not); whether respondent has health insurance	Needs Assessment of New York State Veterans (Vaughan et al., 2011)

Sociodemographic and Service History Characteristics

To reduce respondent burden, sociodemographic and service history characteristics were extracted from administrative data provided by the Air Force Personnel Center (AFPC). These characteristics included gender, race/ethnicity, age, highest level of education, component during active service, retired versus active status, AFSC grouping, grade, number of previous deployments, the operation supported by the respondent's most recent deployment, duration of the respondent's most recent deployment, years since the respondent's return from his or her most recent deployment, total active years in the military, and years since the respondent retired from the Air Force. This information was provided for the entire sample. Thus, Table 3.1 does include exemplars for the variables that we did include on the survey when needed, but our main source of this type of information was personnel records.

4. Survey Results

This chapter provides an overview of the key findings from this analysis. Detailed findings, when not presented here, may be found in Appendix C. The chapter begins by describing those who participated in the survey. It then reports the survey results in the areas of interest: mental health and substance abuse, physical health and medical care, use of mental health services, interpersonal relationships, occupational functioning, financial stability, housing, and evaluation of the AFW2 and AFRCC programs. In general, we report statistics for single variables and provide both a point estimate and confidence intervals around that point estimate. Confidence intervals have a wider range between upper and lower bounds when sample sizes are smaller, and the estimate has less precision.[1]

Participants in the Survey

As noted earlier, skip patterns were used to minimize respondent burden. Approximately 120 items were seen by all participants. Participants were considered to have a "complete" survey if they had completed at least half of these items (459 of 493 entrants did so and are considered "completers"). Thus, our response rate was 53 percent.[2] Some items were seen by all, such as the items assessing PTSD and MDD symptoms, and may be considered essential information. For those items, approximately 6 percent of survey entrants were missing all the items assessing PTSD; likewise, approximately 7 percent of entrants were missing all items assessing MDD. For those who had received and, hence, rated AFW2 services, individual items missing ranged from 5 to 8 percent. Items missing on three general mental health treatment items were also about 7 percent and up to about 8 percent for the employment status item. Of those

---

[1] Confidence intervals (CIs) help convey the uncertainty that is found in any estimate. Their interpretation is as follows: For the 95-percent CIs that we report, if we measured the same variables in the same way from the same population, in 95 percent of those samples our results would fall within the upper and lower bound we report. In cases where our analyses rest on small sample sizes, there is greater uncertainty in our estimates, and our confidence intervals are wider. For analyses with larger sample sizes, our estimates can be more precise, and our confidence intervals may be quite narrow. When we report that groups are "significantly different," the point estimates for the groups are sufficiently different that even taking into account the estimates' uncertainty, the groups are different on that variable.

[2] Readers should be aware that nonresponse bias may still be of concern, but 53 percent compares favorably to other response rates (see, e.g., Baruch, 1999, who reported declines in average response rates over the years such that the average in 1995 was 48.4 percent; Newell et al., 2004, reported similar declines for military surveys). However, a comparison of respondents to nonrespondents based on administrative data available on the population revealed no substantive differences.

who entered the survey and had missing data, 61 percent were missing only one item, while an additional 18 percent were missing two. Approximately 6 percent of *completers* were missing one or more of the items assessing PTSD. Likewise, approximately 3 percent of *completers* were missing one or more of items assessing MDD. For those who had received and, hence, rated AFW2 services, individual items missing ranged from 4 to 7 percent. Missing items on three general mental health treatment items were less than 1 percent and just over 1 percent for the employment status item. Overall, these results show that missing data were not a systematic problem. We did not use imputation for missing data because the problem did not seem to be extensive and because we report primarily univariate statistics for which small amounts of missing data would not be a cumulative problem—as they might be for multivariate analyses.

Given the availability of administrative data on the population of identified Air Force wounded warriors, we were able to compare survey completers with those who did not respond to the survey on a wide array of sociodemographic and service history characteristics to assess any possible nonresponse bias. Population values (proportions and means) were within the limits of the 95 percent confidence intervals around the point estimates for the sample of airmen who completed the survey on all variables except for highest level of education (i.e., college degree or higher), number of years spent on active duty in the military, and age. Airmen with a college degree or higher were slightly overrepresented in the sample of survey completers relative to the larger population. In addition, airmen who completed the survey had spent approximately one more year on active duty in the military and were older than airmen in the larger population by approximately one year. These differences, while statistically significant given our large sample size, were not substantively meaningful. Overall, the sample of survey completers closely resembled the larger population of medically retired and active-duty airmen served by the Air Force Wounded Warrior Program on these administrative variables. Thus, there is little evidence from this analysis to indicate that airmen who answered our survey differed from those who did not. Accordingly, the creation of poststratification weights was deemed unnecessary. See Appendix C for detailed information on the comparison.

Table 4.1 shows the characteristics of those who did respond to our survey. Our participants were largely male, white, married, and enlisted servicemembers, and mostly from the active component. Most, though not all, had been deployed; this reflects AFW2 eligibility, which includes those injured through combat-related activities such as training. The majority of our participants were classified as medically retired.

Benefits eligibility for this population is somewhat complicated. Most active-duty personnel (and reservists/guardsmen on active-duty status) are enrolled in TRICARE

Prime and generally use military treatment facilities,[3] though in some situations they may see civilian providers. Active-duty personnel may also be referred to VHA facilities for certain types of care (such as polytrauma or spinal cord injuries) and may self-refer to Vet Centers for readjustment counseling.[4] Reservists or guardsmen not currently on active-duty status may be eligible for VA health benefits, have health insurance through their own or their spouses' civilian employer, or pay to enroll in TRICARE Reserve Select. Veterans can be eligible for care at VHA facilities, though enrollment is not automatic, and prioritization is variable.[5] Depending on what disability rating they were given by the military when retiring, veterans may also be eligible for a TRICARE variant or be covered by their own or their spouses' employer-based health insurance.

In general, however, active component airmen, reservists and guardsmen, and retirees may be considered to fall within the umbrellas of different, though in some cases overlapping, systems of care: the military treatment facility for active-duty active component, civilian care for reservists and guardsmen, and the Veteran's Health Administration (VHA) system for veterans/retirees. Thus, we created groups to roughly categorize respondents by a variable we refer to as *duty status* and enable exploration of potential differences among the groups, associated as they are with different suites of benefits and resources: active-duty, active component airmen; current reservists and guardsmen; and retirees.

Table 4.1. Respondent Characteristics (N = 459)

Characteristic	n	Percentage
Retired	284	61.9
Male	394	85.8
White	357	77.8
Married	314	68.4
College degree or higher	96	20.9
Enlisted	393	85.6
Component		
Active Duty	320	69.7
Reserve	65	14.26
Guard	73	15.9

[3] For more information on TRICARE variants and eligibility, see http://www.tricare.mil/Welcome/Eligibility.aspx

[4] For more information on Vet Centers, see http://www.vetcenter.va.gov/index.asp

[5] For more information on eligibility for VA medical care, see http://www.va.gov/healthbenefits/apply/veterans.asp. For more information on priority groups, see http://www.va.gov/healthbenefits/resources/priority_groups.asp

Characteristic	n	Percentage
Number of deployments		
0	47	10.2
1	169	36.8
2 or 3	188	41.0
4 or more	55	12.0
Separation pre-2008	86	18.7

	M	SD
Most recent deployment length (months)	4.63	2.82
Years returned from recent deployment	4.19	2.07
Total active years in military (active duty only)	12.38	6.63
Years since most recent AF separation	1.79	2.23
Age	36.38	9.08

NOTES: 17 percent of the population (versus 21 percent of sample) had at least a college degree as their highest level of education.
Mean=11.03 active years in the military among the population (versus 12.38 years for sample).
Mean age=34.87 of population versus 36.38 of sample.
According to data from the AFW2 program, 29 percent of the population indicated a primary disability related to physical injury; 71 percent indicated a primary disability related to a psychiatric diagnosis, namely PTSD (70 percent) or some other psychiatric diagnosis (1 percent).

Mental Health and Substance Abuse

As noted in the previous chapter, many of our population were included in the AFW2 program because of mental health concerns. Information provided by the Air Force Disability Office records, available for 826 members of our population, suggested similarly high rates of PTSD (74 percent) and high rates of depression or related diagnoses (26 percent). Thus, it is not surprising that our survey found that slightly more than three-quarters of respondents screened positive for current (past month) PTSD on the PCL, and three-quarters of respondents screened positive for current (past two weeks) MDD on the PHQ-8. Table 4.2 displays these results in more detail.

Table 4.2. Positive Screens for PTSD and MDD (N = 459)

Condition	N	Percentage	95% CI LL	95% CI UL
Screen positive for PTSD	359	78.2	74.4	82.0
Screen positive for MDD	342	74.5	70.5	78.5

NOTE: CI = confidence interval; LL = lower limit; UL = upper limit.

Given that many of our participants were retired, we examined whether the odds of screening positive for PTSD or MDD declined or increased significantly as a function of the number of months since the airman had retired. Two binary logistic regression models were estimated among the subset of retired airmen (n = 284) to predict screening positive for PTSD and screening positive for MDD; the number of months since retirement served as the sole predictor. These analyses indicated that airmen who had retired less recently (i.e., longer ago) had significantly lower odds of screening positive for PTSD (OR = 0.985, 95-percent CI [0.973, 0.996]). In contrast, the number of months since retirement did not significantly predict the odds of screening positive for MDD (OR = 0.997, 95-percent CI [0.987, 1.007]). To facilitate interpretation of the association between months since retirement and screening positive for PTSD, we computed recycled predictions (Graubard and Korn, 1999; Setodji et al., 2012) to translate the odds ratio into the predicted probability of screening positive for PTSD at one-year intervals. The predicted probabilities of screening positive for PTSD were as follows: Less than one month ago (i.e., 0 months since retirement), 89 percent; one year ago, 87 percent; two years ago, 85 percent; three years ago, 83 percent; and four years ago, 80 percent.

We also examined the extent to which positive screens for PTSD and MDD varied by duty status. Significant differences across the three groups were found for screening positive for PTSD ($\chi^2[2]$ = 16.88, $p < 0.001$) and screening positive for MDD ($\chi^2[2]$ = 13.62, $p < 0.001$). Follow-up pairwise tests revealed that, relative to active-duty airmen, of whom 66 percent screened positive for PTSD, significantly higher proportions of airmen in the Reserve and Guard (90 percent) and retired (82 percent) airmen screened positive (Reserve and Guard versus active duty: ($\chi^2[1]$ = 9.26, $p < 0.01$); retired versus active duty: ($\chi^2[1]$ = 12.66, $p < 0.001$); retired airmen did not differ significantly from airmen in the Reserve and Guard. A similar pattern of results was found with respect to screening positive for MDD, such that airmen in the Reserve and Guard (92 percent) and retired (77 percent) airmen were significantly more likely to screen positive for MDD relative to active-duty airmen (65 percent) (Reserve and Guard versus active duty: ($\chi^2[1]$ = 10.94, $p < 0.001$); retired versus active duty: (64 percent; $\chi^2[1]$ = 6.83, $p < 0.01$). In addition, airmen in the Reserve and Guard were significantly more likely to screen positive for MDD than were retired airmen (Reserve and Guard versus retired: $\chi^2[1]$ = 4.20, $p < 0.05$). Thus, airmen enrolled in the AFW2 program who were still active duty, active component at the time of our survey indicated experiencing fewer and/or less severe symptoms of PTSD or MDD than did airmen who were already retired, or currently in the Reserve and Guard. Figure 4.1 shows the contrast clearly.

Figure 4.1. Positive Screens for PTSD and MDD, by Current Duty Status

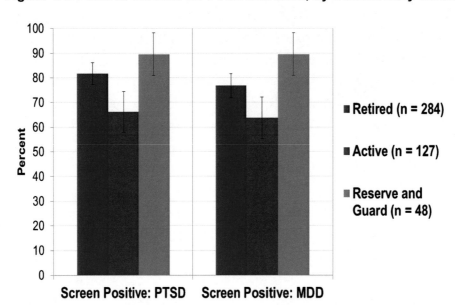

As noted in the literature, PTSD and MDD may often be comorbid with substance use. As shown in Table 4.3, roughly one-quarter of respondents reported that they did not consume any alcohol in the past year. Roughly 40 percent of respondents screened positive for alcohol misuse in the past year based on the AUDIT-C, which is somewhat higher than the roughly 37 percent rate for males and 24 percent rate for females that would be anticipated based on National Epidemiologic Survey on Alcohol and Related Conditions (NESARC) data (i.e., based on general population rates adjusted for the age and gender characteristics of our sample).[6] However, note that the NESARC population estimate for males falls within the confidence intervals of our estimate (lower bound 36 percent, upper bound 45 percent), so the small difference is unlikely to be meaningful. Respondents were also asked about their use of any illicit drugs during the past year.[7]

---

[6] We present age- and gender-adjusted estimates of alcohol misuse in the general population based on NESARC data to provide a point of reference for the interpretation of rates of alcohol misuse in the current sample. There are other factors that are known to affect alcohol misuse (e.g., highest level of education, race/ethnicity) for which no adjustment was made in our comparison estimates. Thus, the comparison of rates of alcohol misuse (and other characteristics and conditions presented subsequently in this chapter, e.g., marital status, unemployment) in the current sample to those in the general population is limited by the lack of adjustment for other relevant factors.

[7] Because alcohol and drug use are particularly sensitive topics to assess in military populations, where known alcohol or drug use can lead to job loss, we expended extra effort to protect the confidentiality of individual responses and to communicate the extent of these protections to respondents prior to their completing the survey. These efforts were designed to safeguard respondents' information to the fullest extent possible and to minimize distortion of reports of alcohol and drug use. We obtained a Certificate of Confidentiality from the National Institute of Mental Health (NIMH), which guards against forced disclosure of data in the event of subpoena. We also implemented a MOU with the Air Force in which the

Specifically, respondents reported on whether they had used marijuana; other illicit drugs such as cocaine, opium, amphetamines, or Ecstasy (MDMA, or 3,4-methylenedioxy-N-methylamphetamine); or prescription medication not prescribed by a physician or taken other than as prescribed. Illicit drug use was much less common than alcohol use, with slightly less than 15 percent of respondents reporting any illicit drug use over the past year. Between 5 and 10 percent of respondents reported use of marijuana or prescription medication other than as prescribed. The reported rates of marijuana use, again, are slightly higher than age- and gender-adjusted rates based on NESARC data, which would lead us to anticipate a rate of 6.8 percent.

Table 4.3. Rates of Alcohol and Illicit Drug Use in the Past 12 Months (N = 459)

Alcohol or Substance Use	N	Percentage	95% CI LL	95% CI UL
Abstinence from alcohol consumption	117	25.5	21.5	29.5
Positive screen for alcohol misuse	187	40.7	36.3	45.2
Any illicit drug use	65	14.2	11.0	17.4
Marijuana use	39	8.5	6.0	11.1
Prescription medication used other than as prescribed	34	7.4	5.0	9.8

NOTE: CI = confidence interval; LL = lower limit; UL = upper limit.

Physical Health and Medical Care

Screening for Traumatic Brain Injury

Given the frequency with which TBI has been found to occur in the combat injured, we screened for this issue. Respondents completed the BTBIS, a brief screener designed to assess whether the individual had experienced an event during deployment or deployment-related activities consistent with a traumatic brain injury. First, respondents were asked whether they had sustained any injuries from a fragment, bullet, vehicular accident, fall, explosion (e.g., improvised explosive device [IED]), or something else. Table 4.4 shows that nearly 90 percent of respondents reported experiencing such a

Air Force agreed not to attempt to reverse-engineer respondents' identities and affirmed understanding of RAND's exclusive ownership of individual-level data. Prospective respondents were informed of these additional layers of protection of confidentiality during the informed consent process prior to deciding whether to participate in the survey. Moreover, survey questions on alcohol and drug use were immediately preceded by a reminder that all responses would be kept confidential. In spite of these efforts, however, it is nonetheless possible that reports of alcohol or drug use are underestimates of the true extent of alcohol and drug use in this population.

deployment-related injury. To determine whether the injury may have been a TBI, respondents were next asked if the injury had resulted in being dazed, confused, or seeing stars; not remembering the injury; or loss of consciousness for any duration. Respondents who reported having experienced an injury with any one of these outcomes were considered to screen positive for the occurrence of a possible TBI. Nearly three-quarters of respondents screened positive for a possible TBI sustained during deployment or related activities. However, it should be kept in mind that a positive screen may not indicate symptoms persistent enough to warrant a medical diagnosis, care, or enduring impairment. Indeed, according to AFW2 program information, the proportion of individuals who are ultimately included in its system for physical injuries on the basis of a TBI overall is relatively small. Moreover, evidence suggests that most individuals who have had a TBI experience an injury that falls into the mild TBI category (Defense and Veterans Brain Injury Center, 2013). In addition, the literature suggests that individuals who experience a mild TBI recuperate fairly soon (within three months to a year), with few persistent effects (see Rohling et al., 2011, for a meta-analytic review).

Table 4.4. Positive Screens for Injuries and Possible TBI Sustained During Deployment or Deployment-Related Activities (N = 459)

Injury	N	Percentage	95% CI LL	95% CI UL
Injury from a fragment, bullet, vehicular accident, fall, explosion (e.g., IED), or something else during deployment or related activities	413	90.0	87.2	92.7
Positive screen for TBI	337	73.4	69.4	77.5

NOTE: CI = confidence interval; LL = lower limit; UL = upper limit.

General Physical Health

We also assessed respondents' physical health using the General Health and Role Limitations based on Physical Health subscales from the SF-36, a well-validated and widely used measure of physical health and functioning (Hays et al., 1993; Ware et al., 1993). Higher scores on the General Health and Role Limitations subscales indicate, respectively, better general health and fewer problems performing work or other activities because of poor physical health. As context for interpretation of scores on these subscales, average (mean) scores were 56.99 (SD = 21.11) on the General Health and 52.97 (SD = 40.78) Role Limitations subscales, in a sample of adult patients with chronic illnesses (hypertension, diabetes, coronary heart disease, and depression) (Hays et al., 1993). As shown in Table 4.5, on average, respondents in our sample had relatively low scores on both subscales, suggesting that they perceive themselves to be in relatively poor health and to have significant role limitations because of physical functioning. However, it is worth noting that respondents' scores on both subscales were variable. Despite relatively low *average* scores on the General Health and Role Limitations subscales, several respondents did report more positive perceptions of their physical health and fewer role limitations due to physical functioning.

Table 4.5. Current Physical Health (N = 459)

Subscale	Mean	Standard Deviation	95% CI LL	95% CI UL
General Health	37.02	24.25	34.8	39.3
Role Limitations due to Physical Health	24.85	33.88	21.7	28.0

NOTES: CI = confidence interval; LL = lower limit; UL = upper limit. General Health and Role Limitations Due To Physical Health are subscales of the SF-36 that were scored according to the RAND method (Hays et al., 1993). For both subscales, possible scores range from 0 to 100, with higher scores on General Health indicating better overall health, and higher scores on Role Limitations due to Physical Health indicating fewer role limitations due to physical health.

Respondents were also asked about their receipt of medical care (any type of care, not just mental health services) from the VA since their return from their most recent deployment or deployment-related activities. Nearly three-quarters of respondents reported having received VA health care since returning from their most recent deployment or deployment-related activities. When asked whether medical care would be helpful, regardless of whether it had been received, nearly all respondents affirmed that it would be helpful. These findings are displayed in Table 4.6. Further information on insurance status and other health-related issues may be found in Appendix C.

Table 4.6. Medical Care Utilization and Desire and Health Insurance Status and Need (N = 459)

	N	Percentage	95% CI LL	95% CI UL
Medical care received at any VA facility since return from most recent deployment or deployment-related activities	339	73.9	69.8	77.9
Medical care would be helpful (regardless of whether it has been received)	428	93.3	91.0	95.5

NOTE: CI = confidence interval; LL = lower limit; UL = upper limit.

Mental Health Services Utilization, Barriers, and Preferences

Given the known mental health concerns of the population as well as the findings regarding current symptoms for mental health conditions, mental health service use is of vital concern for the Air Force's wounded warriors. Respondents were asked a series of questions about their use of mental health services *during the past year*. Of primary interest were those participants who screened positive for PTSD or MDD, or both; these participants made up roughly 83 percent of the sample, or 382 participants. These are the participants whom we have reason to believe have mental health care needs, based on the screeners included in our survey.[8] As shown in Figure 4.2, of those individuals (n = 382), 93 percent received mental health services (i.e., medication, talk therapy, other) for stress, emotional, alcohol, drug, or family problems during the past year), which is quite high. Of those who screened positive for PTSD or MDD and received care (n = 356), 84 percent received both medication and therapy. However, of those who screened positive for PTSD or MDD and received some type of mental health treatment at some point during the past year, approximately half indicated that they had desired professional help at some point in the same time period but had not received it. Thus, despite the high mental health service usage rates observed overall, it appears that the experience of not receiving mental health services at a particular point in time was relatively common. This could include both people who sought care and were unable to get it as well as those who considered seeking care but did not because of an anticipated barrier. Note also that a year is a broad time span, and it is possible that those who reported that they desired care but did not receive it ultimately did get care, just not when they wanted it. The item we used speaks to the perception of lack of access from the airmen's perspective. More detail on the items themselves and overall responses may be found in Appendix C.

Figure 4.2. Service Utilization and Need for Those Who Screened Positive for PTSD or MDD

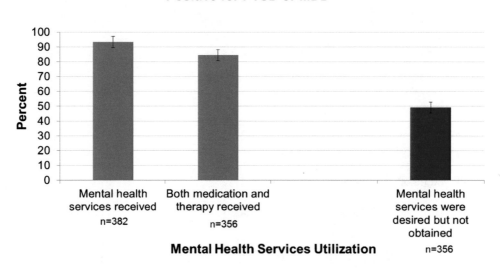

We examined differences in the receipt of any mental health services during the past year and receipt of both medication and therapy compared with only medication, only

---

[8] Note that airmen may also be experiencing mental health symptoms and disorders for which we did not screen. Fewer than five airmen were missing the information on MDD and PTSD; we excluded them from the analyses reported below because we had no information on their mental health needs.

therapy, or neither medication nor therapy across current duty status. There were significant differences across the three groups in receipt of any mental health services during the past year ($\chi^2[2] = 16.81$, $p < 0.001$). Figure 4.3 shows the percentages of airmen of each type of duty status who reported having received mental health services during the past year, for any mental health services and both medication and therapy.

Figure 4.3. Receipt of Past-Year Mental Health Services, by Duty Status

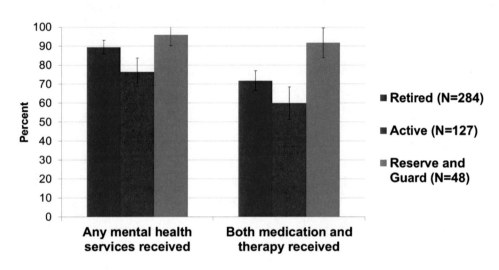

Follow-up pairwise tests of the three groups on the receipt of any mental health services revealed that airmen in the Reserve and Guard and retired airmen were more likely than active-duty airmen to have received mental health services in the past year (retired versus active duty: $\chi^2[1] = 12.00$, $p < 0.001$; Reserve and Guard versus active duty: $\chi^2[1] = 8.82$, $p < 0.01$.) However, receipt of any mental health services during the past year was not significantly more common among airmen in the Reserve and Guard than among retired airmen ($p > 0.05$).

There were also significant differences by duty status in the receipt of both medication and therapy during the past year compared with the receipt of only medication, only therapy, or neither medication nor therapy ($\chi^2[2] = 17.55$, $p < 0.001$). Receipt of both medication and therapy was significantly more common among airmen in the Reserve and Guard relative to retired airmen ($\chi^2[1] = 8.55$, $p < 0.01$) and, in turn, significantly more common among retired airmen relative to active-duty airmen ($\chi^2[1] = 5.81$, $p < 0.05$). These findings may reflect appropriate help-seeking and receipt of services given higher reported symptoms. Our cross-sectional data cannot truly speak to causality, and multiple possibilities exist, including the possibility that the medication and therapy are provided for conditions other than PTSD or other mental health ailment.

Barriers to Treatment

Respondents were asked about several possible barriers to mental health services utilization. Respondents who indicated that there had been a time in the past year when they desired but did not receive mental health services were asked which concerns had prevented them from obtaining professional help.[9] Respondents who indicated that there had *not* been a time in the past year when they desired but did not receive mental health services were asked which concerns would prevent them from seeking professional help if they desired it in the future.

Barriers generally fall into three major categories: logistical, which concerns challenges associated with getting to treatment; institutional and cultural, which refers to concerns about how knowledge of receipt of mental health services could adversely affect one's career or relationships with friends, family, and coworkers if others found out that the airman had received or were currently receiving services; and beliefs about and preferences for treatment.

As shown in Table 4.7, among respondents who had desired help but had not received it at some point in the past year, the most commonly endorsed barriers were concerns about being less respected by friends, family, or coworkers; concerns about the confidentiality of treatment; difficulty scheduling an appointment; concerns about possible harm to one's career; and negative beliefs about the effectiveness of available treatments and side effects of medication. Logistical barriers, such as difficulty identifying a mental health care provider or getting child care or time off of work, were endorsed by approximately one-third of respondents. Cost of care, transportation difficulties, and concerns about loss of contact with or custody of children were the least frequently endorsed barriers, selected by a fifth or less of respondents. Unsurprisingly, respondents who indicated that there had *not* been a time in the past year when they desired but did not receive mental health services, i.e., who did not go without desired help, endorsed the various potential barriers at a far lower rate overall. Their most frequently endorsed barrier was that medications have too many side effects.

---

[9] The actual survey question used to determine whether there had been a time in the past year when respondents desired but did not receive mental health services was: "In the last 12 months, was there ever a time when you wanted to get professional help for stress, emotional, alcohol, drug, or family problems but did not?"

Table 4.7. Barriers to Mental Health Services Utilization (N = 459)

Type of Barrier	Desired help but did not receive it (N = 199)				Did not go without desired help (N = 257)			
	N	Percentage	95% CI LL	95% CI UL	N	Percentage	95% CI LL	95% CI UL
Logistical								
Difficulty scheduling an appointment (VA, MTF, and/or civilian setting)	98	49.3	42.3	56.2	54	21.0	16.0	26.0
Not knowing where to get help or whom to see	69	34.7	28.1	41.3	29	11.3	7.4	15.2
Difficulty getting child care or time off of work	58	29.2	22.8	35.5	47	18.3	13.6	23.0
Difficulty paying for mental health treatment	40	20.1	14.5	25.7	47	18.3	13.6	23.0
Difficulty arranging transportation to treatment	30	15.1	10.1	20.1	27	10.5	6.8	14.3
Institutional and cultural								
Concerns that friends, family, or coworkers would respect airman less	105	52.8	45.8	59.7	40	15.6	11.1	20.0
Concerns about confidentiality of treatment	101	50.8	43.8	57.7	52	20.2	15.3	25.2
Professional help could harm airman's career	96	48.2	41.3	55.2	56	21.8	16.7	26.8
Potential loss of contact or custody of children	27	13.6	8.8	18.3	22	8.6	5.1	12.0
Beliefs about and preferences for treatment								
Perceived ineffectiveness of mental health treatments available to airman	95	47.7	40.8	54.7	60	23.4	18.2	28.5
Medications have too many side effects	90	45.2	38.3	52.1	87	33.9	28.1	39.6
Other reason not mentioned	98	49.3	42.3	56.2	44	17.1	12.5	21.7

NOTES: CI = confidence interval; LL = lower limit; UL = upper limit.

47

The primary focus of intervention is on those individuals who reported a barrier. Thus, we probed further among these respondents, examining whether airmen in the Reserve and Guard, retired airmen, and active-duty airmen differed significantly from each other in their endorsement of barriers to mental health treatment.[10] Although doing so does not isolate the system of care where the problem occurred, given the way we asked the questions, it can help point to the direction of concern. There were three barriers for which there were significant differences by duty status: not knowing where to get help ($\chi^2[2] = 10.67$, $p < 0.01$); concerns that one's friends, family, and coworkers would respect one less ($\chi^2[2] = 9.1$, $p < 0.05$); and concerns about harm to one's career ($\chi^2[2] = 17.77$, $p < 0.001$.) The percentages of airmen of each duty status who endorsed these three barriers are shown in Figure 4.4. There were no significant differences by duty status for any of the other barriers to mental health treatment (all p's > 0.05).

Follow-up pairwise tests to determine which groups differed from each other on the barriers for which there were significant differences indicated that airmen in the Reserve and Guard were more likely to report not knowing where to get help or whom to see for help as a barrier to receiving mental health services than active-duty airmen ($\chi^2[1] = 6.77$, $p < 0.01$) and retired airmen ($\chi^2[1] = 10.43$, $p < 0.01$); active-duty and retired airmen did not differ significantly from each other in their endorsement of this barrier ($p > 0.05$). Follow-up pairwise tests on concerns that others would respect the airman less indicated that airmen in the Reserve and Guard more commonly endorsed this concern than did retired airmen ($\chi^2[1] = 8.08$, $p < 0.01$); airmen in the Reserve and Guard did not differ significantly from active-duty airmen in their endorsement of this concern, nor did active-duty airmen differ significantly from retired airmen in their endorsement of this concern (p's > 0.05). Concerns about harm to one's career were more frequently endorsed by airmen in the Reserve and Guard and active-duty airmen relative to retired airmen (Reserve and Guard versus retired airmen: $\chi^2[1] = 8.47$, $p < 0.01$; active-duty versus retired airmen: $\chi^2[1] = 13.13$, $p < 0.001$). Airmen in the Reserve and Guard did not differ significantly from active-duty airmen in their endorsement of this barrier ($p > 0.05$). Thus, those who were current rather than retired airmen tended to endorse greater cultural and institutional concerns. Additionally, it appears that reservists and guardsmen may experience some confusion regarding resources that they can utilize.

---

[10] Among Airmen who had desired but not received treatment at some point during the past year (n = 199), the cell sizes for current duty status are: retired Airmen (n = 127), active-duty Airmen (n = 49), Reserve and Guard (n = 23).

Figure 4.4. Differences in Mental Health Treatment Barriers, by Current Duty Status (N = 199)

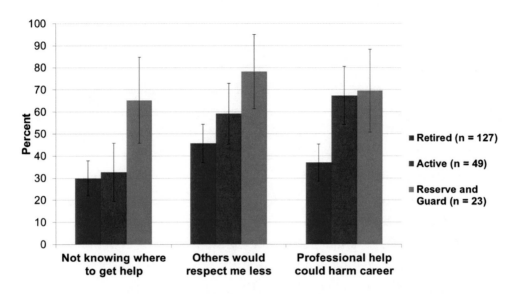

Consideration of barriers invokes the question of *where* these barriers were experienced. In general, active component airmen, reservists and guardsmen, and retirees may be considered to fall under the umbrellas of different though overlapping systems of care: the MTF for active-duty active component, civilian care for reservists and guardsmen, and for our population of veterans with combat-related injuries (note that this includes active-duty airmen as well as reservists and guardsmen, because our sample by definition consists of those with combat-related injuries), the Veterans Affairs Health Administration. However, our analyses show that for airmen in our study strict differentiation by these systems of care did not occur. Relatively comparable proportions of respondents reported having received mental health treatment in a MTF, VHA facility, or civilian facility; roughly half of the respondents had been seen in an MTF or civilian setting, and a little more than half had been treated in a VHA facility (see Table 4.8). In fact, over half of the respondents (52.9 percent; 95-percent CI [48.4, 57.5]) reported having received mental health treatment in two or more types of settings during the past year.

Table 4.8. Mental Health Services Utilization in the Past 12 Months (N = 459)

Mental Health Services Setting	N	Percentage	95% CI LL	95% CI UL
Military treatment facility	221	48.2	43.6	52.7
VHA facility	266	58.0	53.4	62.5
Civilian facility	231	50.3	45.8	54.9

NOTES: CI = confidence interval; LL = lower limit; UL = upper limit; VHA = Veterans Health Administration.

We also explored differences in the settings in which mental health treatment was received during the past year by current duty status to see if this illuminated the systems of care. Table 4.9 shows the percentages of retired airmen, active-duty airmen, and airmen in the Reserve and Guard who were seen by providers in civilian settings, VHA facilities, and MTFs. There were no differences by duty status in receipt of mental health services in a civilian setting ($p > 0.05$). However, there were significant differences by duty status on receipt of mental health services in a VHA facility ($\chi^2[2] = 98.56$, $p < 0.0001$), such that retired airmen and airmen in the Reserve and Guard were more likely than active-duty airmen to report having received mental health services in a VHA facility (retired versus active duty: $\chi^2[1] = 96.42$, $p < 0.0001$; Reserve and Guard versus active duty: $\chi^2[1] = 32.33$, $p < 0.0001$). Retired airmen and airmen in the Reserve and Guard did not differ significantly from each other in the frequency with which they reported having received treatment in a VHA facility ($p > 0.05$). There were also significant differences by duty status on receipt of mental health services in an MTF ($\chi^2[2] = 32.41$, $p < 0.0001$), such that active-duty airmen and airmen in the Reserve and Guard more commonly reported having received treatment in an MTF than retired airmen (active duty versus retired: $\chi^2[1] = 27.0$, $p < 0.0001$; Reserve and Guard versus retired: $\chi^2[1] = 11.83$, $p < 0.001$). Active-duty airmen and airmen in the Reserve and Guard did not differ significantly from each other in the frequency with which they reported having received mental health services in an MTF ($p > 0.05$). However, even with these differences, the evident overlap in systems of care for these respondents makes it difficult to determine the treatment settings to which the barriers reported are most relevant.

Table 4.9. Mental Health Treatment Settings, by Current Duty Status (N = 459)

Current Duty Status	N	Percentage	95% CI LL	95% CI UL
Civilian setting				
Retired (n= 284)	145	51.1	45.2	56.9
Active duty (n = 127)	57	44.9	36.2	53.5
Reserve and Guard (n = 48)	29	60.4	46.6	74.3
VHA				
Retired (n= 284)	208	73.2	68.1	78.4
Active duty (n = 127)	26	20.5	13.5	27.5
Reserve and Guard (n = 48)	32	66.7	53.3	80.0
MTF				
Retired (n= 284)	107	37.7	32.0	43.3
Active duty (n = 127)	83	65.4	57.1	73.6
Reserve and Guard (n = 48)	31	64.6	51.1	78.1

NOTES: CI = confidence interval; LL = lower limit; UL = upper limit; VHA = Veterans Health Administration; MTF = military treatment facility.

Preferred Setting

In addition to asking general questions regarding where care was received, all respondents were asked what their *preferred* setting for mental health treatment would be if cost were not an issue. Given the choice of receiving treatment from a private, civilian provider; a VA facility; an MTF; or none of these options, slightly over half of the respondents expressed a preference for receiving treatment from a private, civilian provider, as displayed in Table 4.10. Just under one-third of the respondents indicated a preference to receive mental health treatment in a VA facility. An MTF was the least commonly chosen setting, selected by just over one-tenth of respondents.

Respondents were also asked what their preferred *type* of mental health treatment would be if cost were not an issue. More than twice as many respondents chose some type of counseling or talk therapy over medication prescribed by a health care provider. Note that this also may be considered to echo the concerns stated by many in the barriers section regarding concerns about medication side effects. Only 10 percent of respondents indicated that they would want neither medication nor therapy.

Table 4.10. Mental Health Services Preferences (N = 459)

	N	Percentage	95% CI LL	95% CI UL
Preferred mental health services setting				
Private, civilian provider	235	51.2	46.6	55.8
VA facility	146	31.8	27.6	36.1
Military treatment facility	52	11.3	8.4	14.2
None of these	10	2.2	0.1	3.5
Preferred type of mental health service				
Some type of counseling or talk therapy provided by a mental health specialist	277	60.4	55.9	64.8
Medication prescribed by a health care provider	111	24.2	20.3	28.1
Neither medication nor therapy	48	10.5	7.7	13.3

NOTES: CI = confidence interval; LL = lower limit; UL = upper limit.

Variation by duty status in preferences for different settings was also examined. There were no differences in preferences for MTFs as a function of duty status, $p > 0.05$. However, there were significant differences in preferences for VHA facilities ($\chi2[2] = 28.99, p < 0.0001$) and for civilian providers ($\chi2[2] = 13.53, p < 0.01$) across duty status. Airmen in the Reserve and Guard and retired airmen were more likely to prefer VHA facilities relative to active-duty airmen (Reserve and Guard versus active duty: $\chi2[1] = 12.66, p < 0.001$; retired versus active duty: $\chi2[1] = 28.59, p < 0.0001$). Conversely, active-duty airmen were more likely than airmen in the Reserve and Guard and retired airmen to prefer civilian providers (active duty versus Reserve and Guard: $\chi2[1] = 7.08, p < 0.01$; active duty versus retired: $\chi2[1] = 12.09, p < 0.01$). Airmen in the Reserve and Guard and retired airmen did not differ significantly from each other in their preferences for VA or civilian providers, p's > 0.05. Provider preferences by duty status are presented in Figure 4.5.

51

Figure 4.5. Preferred Settings for Mental Health Treatment (N = 459)

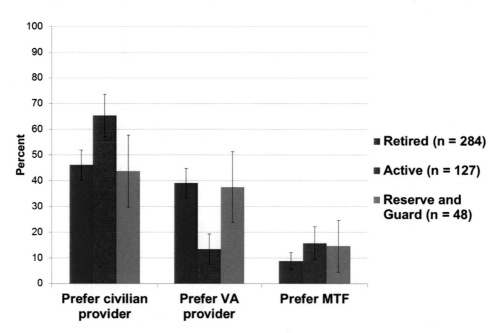

We sought to understand the characteristics of airmen who preferred civilian providers. To this end, we examined the utility of sociodemographic and service history characteristics and perceived barriers to mental health treatment as predictors of civilian provider preferences in a multivariate logistic regression model. We included sociodemographic and service history characteristics and all mental health treatment barriers assessed in the survey as predictors in the model.

The final multivariate regression model included duty status, which was modeled as two dummy variables where retired airmen served as the reference group, officer (versus enlisted), gender, marital status, race/ethnicity modeled as three dummy codes (Hispanic, non-Hispanic black, and non-Hispanic other race/ethnicity) where non-Hispanic white served as the reference group, age, and all of the mental health treatment barriers shown in Table 4.11, which presents results of the final multivariate regression model. As shown, airmen who were active duty (versus retired) and endorsed difficulty paying for mental health treatment, concerns about the effectiveness of available treatments, and concerns about the confidentiality of treatment had significantly greater odds of preferring civilian providers.[11]

---

[11] We also examined the same set of predictors of preferences for civilian providers in the subset of 199 Airmen who reported having desired but not received mental health treatment at some point during the past year. The only predictors that were significant at $p < 0.05$ in this subset of airmen were difficulty paying for mental health treatment (OR = 2.86, 95-percent CI [1.02, 8.00]) and concerns about confidentiality of treatment (OR = 2.41, 95-percent CI [1.08, 5.36]).

To facilitate interpretation of the model results, we computed recycled predictions to translate the odds ratios for each of the statistically significant mental health treatment barriers into the predicted probability of preferring civilian providers among airmen who did and did not endorse the barrier while all other predictors in the model were held constant at their average values. Among airmen who endorsed difficulty paying for mental health treatment, the predicted probability of preferring civilian providers was 0.67 (95-percent CI [0.55, 0.79]); among those who did not endorse difficulty paying for mental health treatment, the predicted probability of preferring civilian providers was 0.49 (95-percent CI [0.43, 0.55]). Among airmen who endorsed concerns about the effectiveness of available treatments, the predicted probability of preferring civilian providers was 0.61 (95-percent CI [0.52, 0.71]); by contrast, among airmen who did not endorse concerns about the effectiveness of available treatment, the predicted probability of preferring civilian providers was 0.48 (95-percent CI [0.41, 0.55]). Among airmen who reported concerns about the confidentiality of treatment, the predicted probability of preferring civilian providers was 0.70 (95-percent CI [0.60, 0.79]); among those who did not endorse this type of concern, the predicted probability of preferring civilian providers was 0.44 (95-percent CI [0.37, 0.51]). These results suggest ongoing concerns regarding the effectiveness of available treatments and the stigma associated with seeking treatment among airmen, particularly those who are active-duty Air Force members. These concerns may drive some of the reported preference for civilian providers.

Table 4.11. Final Multivariate Regression Model Predicting Civilian Provider Preferences (N = 459)

Predictors	OR	95% CI LL	95% CI UL
Active (versus retired)	2.34*	1.41	3.87
Reserve and Guard (versus retired)	0.91	0.43	1.94
Officer	1.71	0.87	3.36
Male	0.63	0.32	1.23
Married	0.68	0.43	1.09
Hispanic (versus white)	0.60	0.29	1.23
Black (versus white)	0.57	0.23	1.40
Other race/ethnicity (versus white)	0.85	0.18	4.11
Age	0.98	0.95	1.01
Not knowing where to go or whom to see	0.97	0.53	1.80
Difficulty arranging transportation to treatment	0.82	0.40	1.66
Difficulty getting child care or time off of work	1.26	0.70	2.28
Difficulty scheduling an appointment	0.94	0.56	1.58
Difficulty paying for mental health treatment	2.09*	1.14	3.82
Concerns that available treatments are not effective	1.72*	1.04	2.83
Medications having too many side effects	0.75	0.46	1.23
Concerns that friends, family, or coworkers would respect airman less	1.33	0.74	2.40
Concerns about confidentiality of treatment	2.98*	1.66	5.35
Concerns about losing contact with or custody of children	0.48†	0.22	1.03
Concerns about harm to professional career	0.81	0.45	1.46
Other reason not mentioned	1.00	0.59	1.67

NOTES: OR = odds ratio; CI = confidence interval; LL = lower limit; UL = upper limit. Note that in some cases, skewed predictor variable proportions may limit the analyses' power to detect significant relationships (e.g., males are far more frequent in our population than females). The two degree-of-freedom joint test of the dummy variables that collectively represented duty status as a predictor in the final multivariate regression model was significant: $\chi^2[1] = 11.47$, $p < 0.01$.
* $p < 0.05$. † $p = 0.06$.

Interpersonal Relationships

Although to some extent information on marital status, number of dependents, etc., represents demographic information and may as such be included in personnel records, these factors are more variable than some of the other demographic information we obtained (i.e., rank at time of separation is unlikely to change, but marital and parental status may change for a number of reasons). Given the large proportion of retirees whose personnel records are not updated, we elected to ask questions regarding these factors in the survey itself. As shown in Table 4.12, the majority of respondents were married. On average, married respondents had been together for roughly 12-and-a-half years. Just over one-fifth of respondents reported that they had no current exclusive relationship. Less than one-tenth of respondents were married and living separately by choice, cohabiting, or dating exclusively. Age and gender adjusted rates based on the November 2011 Census would suggest a population marital rate of 53 percent; thus, respondents from our sample tended to be married more than would otherwise be expected.

Approximately one-third (33.99 percent; 95 percent CI [29.65 percent, 38.32 percent]) reported having no dependent children under the age of 23; only about 15 percent reported living alone (15.47 percent; 95 percent CI [12.16 percent, 18.78 percent]). See Appendix C for other information regarding dependent children and household structure, as well as perceived instrumental and emotional support.

Table 4.12. Current Relationship Status and Length of Current Relationship (N = 459)

Relationship Status	Relationship Status				Relationship Length (years)			
	N	Percentage	95% CI LL	95% CI UL	M	SD	95% CI LL	95% CI UL
Married and living together or living separately due to separate military assignments	285	62.1	57.7	66.5	12.57	8.60	11.57	13.58
Married and living separately by choice	29	6.3	4.19	8.5	10.66	7.42	7.83	13.48
Cohabiting	19	4.1	2.3	6.0	4.43	4.26	2.38	6.49
Dating exclusively	19	4.1	2.3	6.0	1.67	1.35	1.00	2.34
No current exclusive relationship	101	22.0	18.2	25.78	N/A	N/A	N/A	N/A

NOTES: CI = confidence interval; LL = lower limit; UL = upper limit; M = mean; SD = standard deviation; N/A = not applicable.

To determine whom the airmen consider their key source of social support, they were asked to identify the one individual "who most often helps you deal with problems that come up." The airmen were asked to select the relationship of this person to them from a list of response options that included spouse or domestic partner, boyfriend or girlfriend, child, parent/parent-in-law, sibling/sibling-in-law, other relative, a friend, or not applicable (do not share problems with anyone). As shown in Table 4.13, nearly half of respondents selected their spouse or domestic partner as their primary supporter. Just over one-quarter of respondents indicated that they do not have a primary supporter, i.e., they do not share their problems with anyone. Minorities of respondents (i.e., less than 10 percent) named a friend, parent or parent-in-law, other relative, or boyfriend or girlfriend as their primary supporter. Not having an identified primary supporter may be because of a dearth of social support resources or a personal choice not to share problems. Hence, the proportion of respondents reporting this status may or may not consider it a problem that they do not have someone with whom to share. Nonetheless, it may be considered an indicator of potential risk in terms of availability of social support resources.

Table 4.13. Relationship of Primary Supporter to Airman (N = 459)

Relationship	N	Percentage	95% CI LL	95% CI UL
Spouse or domestic partner	214	46.6	42.1	51.2
Not applicable (don't share problems with anyone)	121	26.4	22.3	30.4
Friend	44	9.6	6.9	12.3
Parent/parent-in-law	40	8.7	6.1	11.3
Other relative	19	4.1	2.3	6.0
Boyfriend or girlfriend	15	3.3	1.6	49

NOTES: CI = confidence interval; LL = lower limit; UL = upper limit.

We also assessed whether the absence of a primary supporter, i.e., answering "not applicable (don't share problems with anyone)" in response to the question about the individual to whom one most often turns for help with problems that come up, varied by current duty status. There were no significant differences ($p > 0.05$) among the three groups in the probability of not having a primary supporter.

Respondents were asked to report their level of relationship satisfaction with the individual to whom they were married or, if not married, with the individual identified as their primary supporter. Levels of relationship satisfaction were rated on a scale with response options that ranged from 1 (very dissatisfied) to 5 (very satisfied). Table 4.14 shows respondents' average levels of relationship satisfaction by relationship type. In general, respondents tended to endorse high levels of satisfaction with their marriage or primary supporter. Respondents who were married and living together or living separately as a result of military assignments or who rated their level of satisfaction with their primary supporter had average relationship satisfaction scores that were between a four and a five. Not surprisingly, the one exception to this was respondents who were separated from their spouse; this group's average level of relationship satisfaction was just under two, indicating dissatisfaction with their relationship.

Table 4.14. Average Levels of Relationship Satisfaction with Marriage or Relationship with Primary Supporter (N = 459)

Relationship	N	M	SD	95% CI LL	95% CI UL
Spouse					
Married and living together or living separately due to military assignments	285	4.01	1.24	3.87	4.16
Married and living separately by choice	29	1.59	1.30	1.09	2.08
Primary Supporter					
Live-in domestic partner or boyfriend or girlfriend	21	4.24	0.89	3.83	4.64
Parent/parent-in-law	27	4.41	0.97	4.02	4.79
Other relative	12	4.17	1.19	3.41	4.92
Friend	29	4.66	0.61	4.42	4.89

NOTES: M = mean; SD = standard deviation; CI = confidence interval; LL = lower limit; UL = upper limit. Respondents who were not married and did not identify a primary supporter were skipped out of this question.

Occupational Functioning

Approximately 41 percent of respondents indicated that they were employed full time. While not a majority, this is the single largest group of respondents, as shown in Table 4.15. Fully 25 percent indicated that they were disabled and not working, while the comparative U.S. Bureau of Labor Statistics (BLS) U3 measure of unemployment (i.e., those who are seeking employment out of the total of those who are employed full or part time plus those who are seeking employment) among these wounded warriors is 14 percent. This compares to the age and gender adjusted rate of 8.2 percent for November 2011 (BLS). Eleven percent reported not working by choice, while about 8 percent are pursuing educational attainment.

Table 4.15. Current Employment Status (N = 459)

Current Employment Status	N	Percentage	95% CI LL	95% CI UL
Working full time	189	41.2	36.7	45.7
Disabled and not working	117	25.5	21.5	29.5
Not working and not looking for work (retired, homemaker, or unemployed and not looking for work)	50	10.9	8.0	13.7
Student (full or part time)	39	8.5	6.0	11.1
Unemployed and looking for work	35	7.6	5.2	10.1
Working part time	23	5.0	3.0	7.0
Unemployment rate based on BLS' U3 measure of unemployment	35	14.2	9.8	18.5

NOTES: CI = confidence interval; LL = lower limit; UL = upper limit; BLS = Bureau of Labor Statistics. The category "not working and not looking for work" includes airmen who selected retired, homemaker, or unemployed and not looking for work as their current employment status. The unemployment rate based on the BLS U3 measure of unemployment is calculated as the number of individuals who are unemployed and looking for work divided by the workforce, which includes all individuals who are working full time, working part time, or are unemployed and looking for work.

Note that this analysis includes those airmen who, according to personnel records, are still listed as active component, active duty; we asked all airmen to indicate their self-perceived employment status regardless of personnel record status. Naturally enough, there were significant differences by duty status in whether respondents indicated they were working full or part time versus considering themselves to be primarily occupied in one of the other potential categories ($\chi2[2] = 12.94$, $p < 0.01$) such that active-duty airmen were more likely than retirees to say they were employed (follow-up test $\chi2[1] = 12.91$, $p < 0.001$); other group differences were not significant, $p > 0.05$.

Generally speaking, inclusion of active-duty airmen could be problematic in that it may artificially skew the data toward a lower unemployment rate, given that it includes a group employed by definition. Thus, we also examined employment *excluding* these airmen. Table 4.16 below shows that the unemployment rate is relatively similar whether or not these individuals are excluded, though it compares somewhat more favorably to an age and gender adjusted national unemployment rate that is higher for this subset: 9.8 percent for November 2011 (BLS). It is possible that the similarity of the proportions of airmen who indicate that they are working, whether or not active-duty airmen are included, reflects the uncertainty associated with the process of being boarded and rated for disability among airmen whose mental or physical health is poor enough to warrant enrollment in the AFW2 program (i.e., airmen whose records may indicate that they are actively serving may be told that their current duty is to "get well" or are given relatively light workloads and do not perceive themselves as truly working). We did not ask questions to determine, definitively, why airmen self-identified into a given employment category.

A caveat to consider with regard to higher unemployment rates is that when servicemembers leave the service, higher rates of unemployment are anticipated as a matter of course. Again, by definition, these individuals have lost their employment; and many of the airmen who responded to our survey had relatively recent separation dates. Approximately 18 percent of the airmen were separated in 2010 or 2011 according to personnel records, with about 70 percent of those separation dates 2008 or later.

Table 4.16. Current Employment Status, Excluding Active Duty (N = 332)

Current Employment Status	N	%	95% CI LL	95% CI UL
Working full-time	117	35.2	30.1	40.4
Disabled and not working	101	30.4	25.5	35.4
Not working and not looking for work (retired, homemaker, or unemployed and not looking for work)	35	10.5	7.2	13.9
Student (full or part time)	33	9.9	6.7	13.2
Unemployed and looking for work	22	6.6	3.9	9.3
Working part time	20	6.0	3.5	8.6
Unemployment rate based on BLS U3 measure of unemployment	22	13.8	8.5	19.2

NOTE: CI = confidence interval; LL = lower limit; UL = upper limit; BLS = Bureau of Labor Statistics. The category "not working and not looking for work" includes airmen who selected retired, homemaker, or unemployed and not looking for work as their current employment status. The unemployment rate based on the BLS U3 measure of unemployment is calculated as the number of individuals who are unemployed and looking for work divided by the workforce, which includes all individuals who are working full time, working part time, or are unemployed and looking for work.

Airmen who were working full or part time were asked questions to assess their actual and expected hours worked over the past week as well as about time missed. They were also asked about their overall job performance over the past 28 days, or their *presenteeism*, and their overall job satisfaction. Because there were relatively few airmen who indicated they were working part time, and because absenteeism is calculated as the number of hours worked in comparison to what was anticipated by the employer, we grouped these two categories together for analysis.[12] On a scale that ranges from 0 (worst performance) to 100 (top performance), the average estimate for presenteeism was 68.32. Thus, airmen felt their performance was somewhat above a midrange level of performance over the past 28 days.

The average estimate for absenteeism, or time missed from work, was that airmen lost between five and six hours of work over a seven-day period. That is, on average they worked less than their employers expected them to work over that period of time. Over the course of a year, this level of absenteeism would work out to about 36 days lost, out of the amount of time anticipated by employers (note, however, that this amount could exceed 40 hours per week). Also note that the lower limit of the 95 percent confidence interval is a negative number, indicating that many were working *more* hours than anticipated by their employer. (The number of hours per week anticipated by their employer ranged from 0 to 84; the most common response was 40, which captured 43 percent of those indicating that they worked full time.)

Those airmen who were employed at least part time indicated that, on average, their job satisfaction was midway between very dissatisfied and very satisfied, with a slight bent toward very satisfied. Airmen used the full scale, with approximately 12 percent

---

[12] Part-time and full-time employees did not differ significantly on these variables, *p*'s > 0.05.

indicating they were very dissatisfied, while approximately 18 percent indicated that they were very satisfied. These results for job performance and satisfaction are shown below in Table 4.17.

Table 4.17. Job Performance and Satisfaction (N = 210)

	M	SD	95% CI LL	95% CI UL
Presenteeism	68.32	23.64	65.09	71.55
Absenteeism—past 7-day estimate	5.63	59.35	-2.52	13.78
Job satisfaction	3.27	1.26	3.10	3.44

NOTES: M = mean; SD = standard deviation; CI = confidence interval; LL = lower limit; UL = upper limit. Absolute presenteeism, absolute absenteeism, and job satisfaction were assessed only among airmen who reported that they had a full- or part-time job. Presenteeism and absenteeism may be reported in absolute terms, as raw hours worked and raw performance; and in relative terms, in comparison to other workers. We report absolute numbers here. The range of possible scores for absenteeism is -388 to 388, with higher scores indicating more hours of work lost during the past seven days. The range of observed scores for absenteeism was -80 to 240. The range of possible and observed scores for presenteeism is 0 to 100, with higher scores indicating better perceived job performance. Job satisfaction was rated on a Likert scale that ranged from 1 (very dissatisfied) to 5 (very satisfied).

One-way analyses of variance revealed differences by duty status for presenteeism $F(2, 205) = 7.06$, $p < 0.01$ and post-hoc tests using Bonferroni's correction showed that airmen in the Reserve and Guard ($M = 50.91$ percent, $SD = 34.90$ percent) indicated significantly lower performance while on the job than did active duty ($M = 70.27$ percent, $SD = 23.03$ percent, $p = 0.003$) and retired airmen ($M = 70.44$ percent, $SD = 19.93$ percent; $p = 0.002$). Absenteeism and job satisfaction did not differ by duty status, p's > 0.05. Further information regarding self-perceived work involvement, financial aid for education, and job training appears in Appendix C.

If airmen indicated they were unemployed and looking for work or disabled and not working, they were asked what barriers they perceived to their employment. For ease of presentation, in Table 4.18 we have grouped these notionally into disability-related barriers, concerns about qualifications or skills, disincentives to employment, and "other." The most frequently endorsed barriers were feeling not physically capable, feeling uncomfortable or anxious when thinking about working, and feeling that employers were reluctant to hire them because of their disability, respectively; each one was endorsed by more than half of respondents. Given that the majority of respondents to whom we asked these questions reported that they were disabled and not working, concerns regarding disability status are reasonable and rational and not necessarily an avenue for intervention (such as, for example, self-efficacy training). However, other reported barriers are potentially more tractable avenues for intervention. For example, many felt concern regarding their qualifications; in particular they reported feeling that their deployments put them at a disadvantage compared with their civilian counterparts (42 percent) or that they had a general lack of confidence (42 percent). These concerns could potentially benefit from skills or efficacy interventions. One cultural perception of the disabled as a population, particularly veterans, is that they may exaggerate their condition to get benefits (e.g., McNally, 2003; but see also Ruffing, 2013). That would suggest that a focus on keeping benefits would potentially dissuade these disabled airmen from working. Our findings showed that while some were concerned that employment would cause them to lose benefits, only about 27 percent indicated that loss of financial benefits was a concern. It should also be noted that of those who endorsed one or more barriers, none indicated loss of financial benefits was the *only* concern. The majority endorsed multiple barriers. Of respondents, 53.6 percent indicated that they perceived between two and five barriers to employment; 38.6 percent perceived six or more, indicating that these airmen perceive numerous challenges to employment. Given the highly selected sample, it is reasonable to expect that they are indeed experiencing multiple challenges.

Table 4.18. Perceived Barriers to Employment (N = 152)

Barrier	N	Percentage	95% CI LL	95% CI UL
Disability-related barriers				
Not physically capable	96	63.2	55.5	70.8
No one will hire me because of my injury or disability	87	57.2	49.4	65.1
Concerns about qualifications, skills, or abilities needed for civilian labor market				
I feel uncomfortable or get anxious when thinking about working in the civilian workplace	88	57.9	50.1	65.7
Due to my long and/or multiple deployments, I feel behind compared to my peer civilian counterparts	64	42.1	34.3	50.0
I lack confidence in myself and my abilities	64	42.1	34.3	50.0
I do not have the tools or knowledge to translate my military skills to the civilian workforce	37	24.3	17.5	31.2
Not qualified/lack education	30	19.7	13.4	26.1
Not qualified/lack work history	21	13.8	8.3	19.3
Disincentives to obtain employment				
Would lose financial benefits (e.g., disability benefits)	41	27.0	19.9	34.0
Available jobs don't pay enough	37	24.3	17.5	31.2
Would lose medical benefits	24	15.8	10.0	21.6
Other				
Do not know about available jobs	34	22.4	15.7	29.0
Pursuing an education	34	22.4	15.7	29.0
Family prefers I stay at home	26	17.1	11.1	23.1
Do not have good transportation	15	9.9	5.1	14.6

NOTES: CI = confidence interval; LL = lower limit; UL = upper limit. Barriers to employment were assessed only among those who indicated that they were unemployed and looking for work or disabled and not working.

Financial Stability

We asked several questions to assess respondents' financial situations. These questions are about which household member had primary responsibility for managing the finances, household income, number of household members supported by income, and questions to assess perceived financial strain. As with employment, it makes sense to consider estimates for some of these variables that exclude active-duty active component airmen, who may skew the data because they are receiving employment income by definition. We provide both total numbers and numbers with that exclusion, which show relatively little difference, as shown in Table 4.19.

Table 4.19. Financial Resources and Responsibilities

Financial Indicators	Total Sample (N=459)				Excluding AD (N=332)			
	N	Percentage	95% CI LL	95% CI UL	N	Percentage	95% CI LL	95% CI UL
Household income before taxes in 2010								
Less than $30,000	78	17.0	13.5	20.4	59	17.8	13.6	21.9
$30,000 to less than $50,000	140	30.5	26.3	34.7	99	29.8	24.9	34.8
$50,000 to less than $75,000	103	22.4	18.6	26.3	74	22.3	17.8	26.8
$75,000 to less than $100,000	55	12.0	9.0	15.0	41	12.4	8.8	15.9
$100,000 or more	58	12.6	10.0	15.7	43	13.0	9.3	16.6
Number of people in household supported by total household income								
1	90	19.6	16.0	23.2	66	19.9	15.6	24.2
2 or 3	181	39.4	35.0	43.9	133	40.1	34.8	45.4
4 or more	174	37.9	33.5	42.4	124	37.4	32.1	42.6
Below the 2010 HHS federal poverty guidelines	47	10.2	7.5	13.0	35	10.5	7.2	13.9
Person with primary responsibility for managing finances [a]								
Respondent	222	48.4	43.8	52.9				
Spouse or partner	132	28.8	24.6	32.9				
Spouse/partner and respondent share responsibility for finances	83	18.1	14.6	21.6				
	M	SD			M	SD		
Financial strain	2.54	1.22	2.43	2.66	2.53	1.21	2.40	2.66

NOTES: CI = confidence interval; LL = lower limit; UL = upper limit; M = mean; SD = standard deviation; AD= active duty, active component. Number of people in household supported by total household income includes the respondent. Possible and observed scores on the Financial Strain scale range from 1 to 5, with higher scores indicating greater perceived financial strain.
[a] These numbers do not sum to 100 percent due to a few individuals marking other responses.

The Census Bureau reported that median household income in the United States in 2010, the year for which our respondents reported income, was $49,445. About 53 percent of the respondents indicated that their household income fell between $30,000 and $74,999. Of our total sample of airmen, the largest number of respondents (30.50 percent) indicated that their income fell between $30,000 and $50,000 (similarly, excluding active-duty airmen yielded a modal frequency of 29.82 percent). About one-quarter, 24.62 percent (excluding active duty, 25.30 percent), indicated that their income was at least $75,000. Approximately 10 percent of respondents *might be* at risk of falling below Department of Health and Human Services (HHS) poverty guidelines, based on the number of individuals who were supported by their 2010 household income. HHS poverty guidelines are used to determine eligibility for certain federal aid programs and are not the same as the poverty thresholds reported by the Census Bureau. Moreover, this is a rough categorization based on the categorical nature of how household income was reported in our survey. For example, the guideline for a household of two people in the contiguous United States is $14,570 in household income; however, we coded someone as "at risk" if a household of two people was supported by anything less than $20,000. Thus, our "at risk" categorization is more inclusive than the poverty guidelines. The figures once active-duty airmen have been excluded are largely similar; over 50 percent of the retirees and those in Reserve and Guard who reported income indicated that theirs fell between $30,000 and $74,999.

Although a comparatively low proportion of airmen responded in a manner consistent with falling below HHS's poverty guidelines, the question then becomes: What level indicates a need for intervention? This is a matter for policymakers to decide, but the nature of our population may suggest that even a comparatively low rate is potentially a matter for concern and intervention.

Almost half of respondents indicated that they had primary responsibility for household finances, and another 20 percent or so indicated that they shared these responsibilities with a partner.

Respondents were asked three questions to assess perceived financial strain; each question was rated on a 1 to 5 scale with higher scores indicative of greater perceived strain. These questions explored difficulty living on income; whether there was a perceived need to cut expenses to the minimum; and whether the participant perceived a risk of going without food, shelter, or other necessities. On average, the distribution of respondents fell at the lower end of the range, suggesting that they perceived relatively little financial strain. However, the full distribution was used, which indicates that some airmen did perceive higher levels of strain.

Housing Instability

Risk factors for homelessness include a history of housing instability (Koegel, 2004). Thus, we asked airmen whether they had ever spent the night in one of the following locations: a transitional shelter or program, a homeless shelter, in a chapel or church (but not in a bed) an all-night theater or other indoor public place, an abandoned building, a car or vehicle, or the street or other outdoor place, because they had no regular place to stay. As shown in Table 4.20, among airmen, about one-fifth had spent the night in one of these locations, which indicates possible homelessness. A previous survey question had asked airmen how long it had been since they returned from their most recent deployment. In this section, we asked them how recently they had stayed in a location indicative of possible homelessness and then compared that date with the date of their return from deployment. Just over 10 percent indicated that they had been in such a situation since their return, and over 9 percent indicated that their *first* experience in such a situation occurred since their return. On average, respondents indicated that it had been just under eight years since they had last spent the night in such a setting.

Table 4.20. Lifetime History of Homelessness (N = 459)

	N	Percentage	95% CI LL	95% CI UL
Ever spent the night homeless	99	21.6	17.8	25.3
Homeless since return from most recent deployment	48	10.5	7.7	13.3
First time homeless occurred since return from most recent deployment	43	9.4	6.7	12.0
	M	**SD**	**95% CI LL**	**95% CI UL**
Years since spent last night in homeless setting	7.88	10.01	5.76	10.00

NOTES: CI = confidence interval; LL = lower limit; UL = upper limit; M = mean; SD = standard deviation. Homeless is defined as a report of spending the night in one of the following due to no regular place to stay: (1) a transitional shelter or program, (2) a homeless shelter, (3) in a chapel or church (but not a bed), (4) in an all-night theater or other indoor public place, (5) an abandoned building, (6) a car or vehicle, or (7) the street/other outdoor place.

Only those who had ever spent the night in a potentially homeless setting were asked the subsequent questions, because we assumed anyone *currently* in a setting indicative of homelessness would logically be a subset of this group. For these individuals, we wanted to assess their housing situation in greater detail. First, we asked them how long they had lived at their current place of residence; on average, airmen had been at their current residence three and one-half years. Forty-one percent of this subset of respondents had lived at only one location within just the past six months, while 59 percent had lived in two or more different locations. One-fifth had lived in four or more locations, indicating quite a bit of mobility over a six-month period. Figure 4.6 makes clear, however, that many respondents had lived in a small number of locations for the prior six months.

Figure 4.6. Number of Different Residence Locations Within the Past Six Months

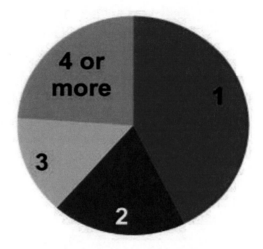

NOTE. This figure includes only the subset of airmen who indicated that they had ever spent the night in a potentially homeless setting.

We wanted to parse the character of the number of different housing situations respondents had within the past six months in greater detail than we had for our screener item. We therefore asked respondents if they had spent the night in a wide variety of locations during that time and included in particular a greater breadth of detail on housing situations that might be considered "homeless." Table 4.21 describes the variety of potential housing situations that respondents could choose from, and our classification of that housing situation (i.e., how we categorized it). Note that our classification system echoes the current legislative framework in characterizing residence in voucher-paid locations as homelessness.

Table 4.21. Classification of Housing Situation Options

Classification	Housing Situation
Not homeless	Their own home or a partner's home
At-risk for homelessness	• Home of family or friends • Hotel paid for by self, partner, or family or friends • Residential alcohol or drug detox • Psychiatric hospital or drug treatment facility • Hospital
Homeless	• Hotel or motel room paid for with a voucher • Boarding, transition or halfway house • Mission or shelter • Church or chapel • All-night theater or similar • Abandoned building • Vehicle • Street

As can be seen in Figure 4.7, about one-third (33 percent) indicated that they spent time in a housing situation that we classify as "homeless" in the past six months. This works out to about 7 percent of our total respondents, keeping in mind that only airmen who had a past experience of potential homelessness were even asked these questions. An additional 23 percent would be considered "At risk" (5 percent of 459).

Figure 4.7. Housing Situation in Prior Six Months of Airmen with Lifetime History of Homelessness

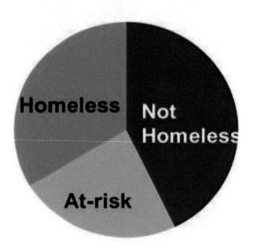

We also asked airmen about other aspects of their housing situation during the prior six months. The figures for those who did respond to these targeted questions can be seen in Table 4.22. When asked how long they spent in such a setting, the response was on average about one month, although the reported range varied widely from two to 180 days. We also asked airmen whether *they considered themselves* to have been homeless within the past six months; given the wide variety of settings we asked about and the equally wide variety of potential reasons for being in some of these settings, we felt this self-perception was important. However, it should also be noted that being homeless is stigmatized in our society, and so individuals who have experiences that would classify them as homeless from an external perspective may or may not classify *themselves* as such. About 18 percent of the subset that answered these questions indicated that they considered themselves to have been homeless in the past six months. This works out to only about 4 percent of all airmen who responded to our survey, since as noted above, most of our respondents indicated no lifetime history of potential homelessness. We also asked about current living situation, and found that 17 percent of airmen with a lifetime history of potential homelessness indicated that, at the time they responded to the survey, they were currently living in a situation that fell into our "at risk" or "homeless" categorizations.

Table 4.22. Self-Reported Housing Situation During the Past Six Months of Airmen with a Lifetime History of Potential Homelessness (N = 99)

	M	SD	95% CI LL	95% CI UL
Number of years respondent has been living in current place of residence	3.53	6.14	2.30	4.77
Number of days spent homeless during the past 6 months	31.32	48.72	9.72	52.92

NOTES: M = mean; SD = standard deviation; CI = confidence interval; LL = lower limit; UL = upper limit.

We also asked airmen about some potential remedies to housing difficulties. About 20 percent of airmen received some form of housing assistance since their return from deployment or since their deployment-related activities, as shown in Table 4.23. However, a large majority (approximately 75 percent) indicated that they perceived such assistance to be potentially helpful. Moreover, almost half of airmen felt that transitional housing would be helpful, although fewer than ten had taken advantage of such assistance since their return.

Perceived helpfulness of housing assistance or loans differed significantly by duty status ($\chi^2(2) = 7.98$, $p < 0.05$). Follow-up pairwise tests indicated significant differences between retired airmen and airmen in the Reserve and Guard ($\chi^2(1) = 7.90$, $p < 0.01$), such that retired airmen more commonly perceived that housing assistance or loans would be helpful (78.52 percent; 95-percent CI [73.74, 83.30]) than did airmen in the Reserve and Guard (58.33 percent; 95-percent CI [44.39, 72.28]). There were no significant differences between active-duty airmen (73.23 percent; 95-percent CI [65.53, 80.93]) and retired airmen or airmen in the Reserve and Guard (p's > 0.05). Housing adjustment is different for airmen in the Reserve and Guard, who are able to return to their hometowns after deployment; active component airmen do not need to move unless they are reassigned and, moreover, have access to military housing options. Thus, the most dramatic housing adjustment is for medically retired, and this fact appears to be reflected in our findings.

Table 4.23. Housing Resources That Have Been Received or Would Be Helpful (N = 459)

	N	Percentage	95% CI LL	95% CI UL
Housing assistance or loans received since return from most recent deployment or deployment-related activities	83	18.1	14.6	21.6
Housing assistance or loans would be helpful	344	75.0	71.0	78.9
Transitional housing would be helpful	213	46.4	41.8	51.0

NOTES: CI = confidence interval; LL = lower limit; UL = upper limit. The housing resources listed in the table are available to combat-injured airmen and veterans.

Program Evaluation

Air Force Wounded Warrior Program

Nearly all respondents reported that they had been in contact with a representative of the AFW2. The great majority of respondents reported that they had initially been contacted by the AFW2 representative. Recall that we drew our sample from the population of AFW2 enrollees, so this high level of contact is unsurprising.

Respondents were asked to indicate which of several types of services or help offered by AFW2 they had received from an AFW2 representative. Nearly all (roughly 95 percent) respondents indicated that they had received at least one type of service or help, suggesting that the AFW2 program has achieved a high rate of penetration among its enrollees (see Table 4.24). Each type of service assessed had been used by at least half of respondents. The types of AFW2 services that had been received by respondents were, from most to least frequently endorsed, regular supportive calls (89 percent), help or advice for filling out paperwork (73 percent), contact from someone providing assistance at the request of AFW2 (71 percent), referrals to other services (64 percent), advice for life matters (57 percent), and advice for dealing with red tape (53 percent). More than half of respondents (59 percent) indicated having received some other type of service of an unknown nature. The finding that regular supportive calls, the most commonly received type of service, were received by the great majority of respondents suggests that the AFW2 program functions as a source of social support for its clients.

Table 4.24. Air Force Wounded Warrior Program Utilization (N = 459)

	N	Percentage	95% CI LL	95% CI UL
Contact with AFW2 representative	453	98.7	97.7	99.7
AFW2 representative initiated contact first	395	86.1	82.9	89.2
Regular supportive calls	410	89.3	86.5	92.2
Help or advice for filling out paperwork	336	73.2	69.2	77.3
AFW2 representative had someone contact the airman to provide assistance	324	70.6	66.4	74.8
Referrals to other services	292	63.6	59.2	68.0
Advice for life matters	262	57.1	52.6	61.6
Advice for dealing with red tape	241	52.5	47.9	57.1
Some other type of service	271	59.0	54.5	63.5
Received at least one type of service	437	95.2	93.3	97.2

NOTES: CI = confidence interval; LL = lower limit; UL = upper limit. Received at least one type of service means that the respondent indicated having received one or more of the following services: referrals to other services, help or advice for filling out paperwork, advice for life matters, advice for dealing with red tape, contact from someone who gave assistance, regular supportive calls, or some other type of help or service.

Respondents who reported having received at least one type of service or help from an AFW2 representative were subsequently asked whether they agreed or disagreed with several statements designed to assess their perceptions of specific services provided by AFW2 and their overall satisfaction with the program. As shown in Table 4.25 below, the vast majority of respondents agreed that AFW2 case managers are available and ready to help (92 percent) and provide good information on available resources (89 percent), indicating that these aspects of the program are strengths. Nearly three-quarters of respondents perceived that services available through AFW2 case managers can help with issues caused during the respondent's service in the Air Force. Thus, confidence in the actual services provided, although expressed by the majority of respondents, was slightly less widespread than confidence in the AFW2 case managers themselves. Just over one-quarter of respondents agreed that they would like to be contacted by AFW2 case managers more often, indicating that the majority of respondents do not perceive the need to increase contact with AFW2 case managers. Finally, when asked if they were satisfied overall with services provided by the AFW2 program, the great majority of respondents (86 percent) affirmed their overall satisfaction. Overall satisfaction with AFW2 services and number of positive statements endorsed did not differ significantly by duty status ($p > 0.05$). In sum, although there were some respondents who expressed dissatisfaction with different aspects of the AFW2 program, satisfied program users were much more heavily represented in this sample than were dissatisfied program users.

Table 4.25. Air Force Wounded Warrior Program Perceptions (N = 437)

Perception	N	Percentage	95% CI LL	95% CI UL
AFW2 case managers are available and ready to help	403	92.2	89.8	94.7
Case managers provide good information on available resources	389	89.0	86.1	92.0
Services available through AFW2 case managers can help with issues caused during AF service*	321	73.5	69.3	77.6
Would like to be contacted by AFW2 case managers more often	116	26.5	22.4	30.7
Overall satisfied with services provided by AFW2 program	375	85.8	82.5	89.1

NOTES: CI = confidence interval; LL = lower limit; UL = upper limit. The denominator for these descriptive statistics was limited to respondents who reported having used at least one service to ensure that respondents would have at least some relevant experience to inform their assessment of the AFW2 program. The frequencies and percentages reflect how many respondents agreed with the AFW2 program perception listed in the left-hand column. The asterisk (*) marks a statement that was negatively worded in the survey, i.e., the respondent was asked whether he/she agreed or disagreed that "The services available through AFW2 case managers can't really help me deal with any issues caused during my Air Force service."

We also sought to identify the characteristics of airmen who expressed the desire to be contacted by AFW2 case managers more often. To this end, we estimated a multivariate model to predict the desire for more frequent contact with AFW2 case managers. The multivariate model included several sociodemographic and service history characteristics and theoretically meaningful predictors that represent risk in the domains that we examined. Predictors in the final model included the number of months since retirement, duty status (represented as two dummy codes for active duty, active component, and Reserve and Guard with retired as the reference category), officer (versus enlisted), gender, marital status, age, race/ethnicity (represented as three dummy codes for Hispanic, non-Hispanic black, and non-Hispanic other where white was the reference category), screening positive for PTSD, general health, role limitations due to physical health, screening positive for TBI, financial strain, lifetime history of homelessness, and current employment status. The only predictors that were significant at $p < 0.05$ in the final model were Hispanic (versus white) (OR = 2.77, 95-percent CI [1.35, 5.67]) and general health (OR = 0.99, 95-percent CI [0.98, 0.999]).[13] Thus, Hispanic airmen and airmen with poorer physical health had significantly higher odds of desiring more frequent contact with AFW2 case managers. To interpret these effects, we computed recycled predictions to convert the odds ratios to predicted probabilities of desiring more frequent contact with AFW2 case managers among Hispanics and non-Hispanics and airmen with various levels of self-reported physical health while holding all other predictors in the model constant at their average values. The predicted probabilities of desiring more frequent contact with AFW2 case managers were 46 percent for Hispanics and 24 percent for non-Hispanics. Across the range of physical health self-ratings, the predicted probabilities of desiring more frequent contact with AFW2 case managers were: excellent health, 13 percent; very good health, 17 percent; good health, 23 percent; fair health, 29 percent; poor health, 36 percent. Note that our cell sizes for this analysis were quite small, which may render the findings unstable; we suggest interpreting this finding such that airmen with characteristics found in the literature to be related to greater vulnerability overall (minority status, poor health; see, e.g., Karney et al.'s 2008 discussion of the stress-diathesis model) may have a greater desire for contact from care providers.

Air Force Recovery Care Coordinator Program

Respondents were asked about their use of services offered by the AFRCC program and their perceptions of the program. Table 4.26 shows that slightly less than a fifth of respondents reported having received any help or services from the AFRCC program. Nearly twice as many respondents were unsure of what the AFRCC program is, and more than twice as many respondents indicated not having received help or services from the

---

[13] The two degrees-of-freedom joint test of significance for race/ethnicity, as represented by the two dummy-coded variables Hispanic and black/African American (with white as the reference group), was significant at $p < 0.05$: $\chi^2(2) = 8.01$.

AFRCC program. Thus, a minority of respondents had used the AFRCC program. This should not be taken as a cause for concern, however, because the eligibility requirements for the AFRCC program include significant injuries, whether combat related or not. Moreover, the program itself did not begin rollout prior to 2008, and rollout was phased throughout that year. Thus, while some overlap in services was anticipated, a one-to-one correspondence of the AFW2 population with AFRCC was not expected.

Table 4.26. Air Force Recovery Care Coordinator Program Utilization (N = 459)

Help or Services Received from AFRCC Program[a]	N	Percentage	95% CI LL	95% CI UL
Yes	91	19.8	16.2	23.5
No	189	41.2	36.7	45.7
Not sure what AFRCC program is	170	37.0	32.6	41.5

NOTES: CI = confidence interval; LL = lower limit; UL = upper limit.
[a] Fewer than 10 individuals indicated that the program was "not applicable."

As displayed in Table 4.27, the most commonly used AFRCC services were referrals to other services and programs for veterans or combat-injured airmen and help accessing these services and programs. These findings suggest that a key function of the AFRCC program is facilitating access to services and programs for veterans or combat-injured airmen. Regular supportive calls were another frequently utilized service, indicating that, like the AFW2 program, the AFRCC program functions as a source of social support for many of its users. Other, somewhat less frequently utilized services or types of help included advice for life matters, help adjusting to or coping with physical or mental health conditions that developed during or after military service, and assistance with goal-setting and planning through the development of a Comprehensive Recovery Plan or Recovery Care Plan; each type of help was received by roughly 55 percent of respondents. Follow-up after the development of the Comprehensive Recovery Plan or Recovery Care Plan was the least commonly received type of service (roughly 53 percent of respondents). However, examination of the subsequent table of service perceptions (Table 4.28) suggests that this endorsement rate may be an issue of airmen perception and "branding" rather an issue of fidelity to the recovery care coordination service plan.

Table 4.27. Air Force Recovery Care Coordinator Program Services Utilized (N = 91)

Services Utilized	N	Percentage	95% CI LL	95% CI UL
Referrals to other services and programs for veterans or combat-injured airmen	74	81.3	73.3	89.3
Help accessing services and programs for veterans or combat-injured airmen	71	78.0	69.5	86.5
Regular supportive calls	66	72.5	63.4	81.7
Advice for life matters	55	60.4	50.4	70.5
Help adjusting to or coping with physical or mental health conditions that developed during or after military service	52	57.1	47.0	67.3
Assistance with goal-setting and planning through the development of a Comprehensive Recovery Plan or Recovery Care Plan	51	56.0	45.9	66.2
Follow-up after the development of Comprehensive Recovery Plan and Recovery Care Plan to help airman stay on track to meet his/her goals	48	52.8	42.5	63.0
Some other help or service	57	62.6	52.7	72.6

NOTES: CI = confidence interval; LL = lower limit; UL = upper limit. Questions about specific AFRCC services utilized were asked only of respondents who had reported receiving help or services from the AFRCC program.

As with the AFW2 program, respondents who reported having received at least one type of help or service from the AFRCC program were asked whether they agreed with statements intended to assess their satisfaction with services received. As shown in Table 4.28, all statements about satisfaction with help received were endorsed in a positive direction by the majority of respondents, indicating that program users tended to be more satisfied than dissatisfied with services received from the AFRCC program. In particular, Recovery Care Coordinators (RRCs) were perceived to be knowledgeable about available resources and highly accessible by the great majority of respondents (87 percent). RCCs were also widely recognized by program users as capable facilitators of access to needed programs and services (80 percent) and achievement of personal goals (76 percent). As recording and achieving of personal goals is one of the hallmarks of a Comprehensive Recovery Plan, this suggests that many airmen do feel that they are receiving the service, although they may not relate it to the program terminology. A slightly lower proportion (68 percent) of program users agreed that RCCs can help with issues or problems caused during the respondent's Air Force service. Roughly three-quarters of respondents affirmed their overall satisfaction with services provided by the AFRCC program.[14]

---

[14] We considered examining differences in satisfaction with the AFRCC program services by current duty status. However, the breakdown of total AFRCC users by current duty status produced very small cell sizes, particularly in the Reserve and Guard, which yielded very unstable estimates and precluded sufficiently powerful tests to examine these differences.

Table 4.28. Air Force Recovery Care Coordinator Program Perceptions (N = 91)

Perception	N	Percentage	95% CI LL	95% CI UL
RCCs can give good information on available resources	79	86.8	79.9	93.8
RCCs are easy to reach	79	86.8	79.9	93.8
RCCs can facilitate access to needed programs and services	73	80.2	72.0	88.4
RCCs can help achieve personal goals	69	75.8	67.0	84.6
RCCs can help with issues or problems caused during AF service*	62	68.1	58.6	77.7
Overall satisfied with services provided by the AFRCC program	68	74.7	65.8	83.7

NOTES: CI = confidence interval; LL = lower limit; UL = upper limit. The denominator for these descriptive statistics was limited to respondents who reported having used at least one service to ensure that respondents would have at least some relevant experience to inform their assessment of the AFRCC program. The frequencies and percentages reflect how many respondents agreed with each of the AFRCC program perceptions listed in the left-hand column. The asterisk (*) marks a statement that was negatively worded in the survey, e.g., the respondent was asked whether he/she agreed or disagreed that "RCCs can't really help me deal with any issues or problems caused during my Air Force service."

AFRCC program users were also asked about concerns regarding possible adverse effects of program use, as shown in Table 4.29. Specifically, program users were asked whether others would think less of them for getting help from the AFRCC program and whether obtaining help would harm their careers. Each concern was endorsed by close to roughly one-fifth of respondents—a nontrivial proportion. Thus, concerns about the possible adverse effect of receiving help on others' perceptions of the respondent and the respondent's career were salient to some respondents.

Table 4.29. Potential Concerns about AFRCC Services Utilization (N = 91)

Barrier	N	Percentage	95% CI LL	95% CI UL
Others (family members, friends, or coworkers) would think less of airman for getting help from AFRCC program	18	19.8	11.6	29.8
Career would be harmed by getting help	19	20.9	12.5	29.2

NOTES: CI = confidence interval; LL = lower limit; UL = upper limit.

To summarize the Program Evaluation section, we asked questions regarding use of and satisfaction with two Air Force programs available to help these airmen. High numbers of respondents indicated that they were receiving services, particularly for the AFW2 program. This is heartening because our population consisted of enrollees in that program. Respondents were also receiving a number of services and reported overall very high levels of satisfaction with the program. Although eligibility requirements and program existence dictated that a smaller proportion of our population would be covered by the AFRCC program, airmen who reported receipt of AFRCC services received a variety and were very satisfied with the program. For both programs, the nature of services provided can be characterized as a form of social support.

5. Conclusions and Recommendations

Our study examined the status of airmen in the fall of 2011 and the support airmen received during that time. We examined well-being based on a number of indicators among a population identified by the Air Force as experiencing reintegration challenges severe enough to warrant consideration for medical retirement because of combat-related injuries and illnesses. Our investigation is somewhat unusual. On the one hand, we attempted to answer the Institute of Medicine's (2010) call for a more sophisticated and holistic examination of reintegration, and hence include measures in domains including mental and physical health, mental health treatment and potential barriers, social support and household structure, employment and financial considerations, and housing instability. We also examined service usage and satisfaction with two Air Force programs emplaced to help airmen deal with some of the challenges we describe. On the other hand, our holistic approach is applied to a highly select population of airmen who have been identified as having injuries and illnesses that are related to combat and hence are in a situation in which their personal resources may already be stretched because of the known challenges they are experiencing. Many programs are in place to help these wounded warriors; we examine in detail only two. Full exploration of the myriad resources is beyond the scope of this, or likely any, single research project (note that the National Resource Directory, an online depository of such resources, lists over *14,000* potential resources, programs, and charities). Consideration of our findings and recommendations must take into account both the time frame of our study and the fact that the Air Force and the many others who serve this important population have been working diligently to improve these programs.

Our results demonstrate that our sample is indeed experiencing challenges in a number of domains. A high proportion of airmen screened positive for PTSD (roughly 78 percent) and MDD (roughly 75 percent); with 69 percent screening positive for both. We also found evidence of somewhat elevated rates of reported substance use and lower rates of perceived physical health within our sample. Although our sample reported very high rates of mental health treatment within the past year for those who needed it (90 percent), within that same time frame about half reported at least one instance when they desired but did not obtain mental health treatment. A one-year time frame is broad. However, given the evident and identified need for mental health services among this population, and the efforts that have been undertaken to tend to servicemembers' mental health needs more effectively, unmet need for mental health treatment remains a pertinent issue. Although not many airmen responded in a manner consistent with falling below HHS's poverty guidelines, about 10 percent could be considered to fall below this guideline.

Similarly, close to 15 percent of our sample would be considered unemployed based on the BLS's oft-reported U3 measure of unemployment. Housing instability represents another potential area of concern, with almost 10 percent of the entire sample indicating that their first experience with housing instability occurred after their return from their most recent deployment.

In brief, the wounded, ill, and, injured airmen in our analysis reported challenges in multiple domains. We focus our recommendations on two of the domains in which problems were notably elevated and that a relatively robust evidence base indicates are potentially amenable to intervention: mental health and employment. These areas are also good ones to focus on because both domains offer opportunities for Air Force nonmedical case managers, whose programs we did evaluate, to assist in the implementation and coordination throughout the continuum of care. Although the scope of this report is necessarily limited to recommendations that the Air Force might implement, others such as the VA and community organizations may find them useful as well. Finally, mitigating concerns in these areas would be expected to have a positive effect on problems in other domains.[1] In the remainder of this chapter, we discuss key findings on barriers to accessing mental health treatment and obtaining employment and offer recommendations for improving outcomes in the domains of mental health and employment. Before delving deeply into these recommendations, we first offer caveats for general consideration as well as a brief discussion of implemented changes in the second wave of the survey.

Brief Caveats

Limitations of our research include its current cross-sectional nature, which restricts the inferences regarding causality that may be drawn from these data. However, as the overall project design is a longitudinal effort, future surveys will help to alleviate this concern. Our sample and population may also be considered a limitation in the sense that it is very select; we included only enrollees in the AFW2 program. As there may be some wounded airmen who are eligible for but not enrolled in the AFW2 program, our results may not generalize to the broader population of wounded airmen. Moreover, as a high percentage of our population had a primary diagnosis of mental health distress rather than physical injury, they may not be representative of the service population with combat injuries, many of whom may have a primary diagnosis of physical injuries. In some cases, our analyses were limited by small sample sizes, which may raise questions about

---

[1] For example, improving employment outcomes would likely promote housing stability (see e.g., Apicello 2010's discussion of individual and structural homelessness prevention efforts. Certainly, maintaining employment is related to maintaining an adequate household income.

the stability of the estimates we obtained. To the extent that our findings reflect the larger literature, some of this concern is alleviated; however, small cell sizes do remain a concern. A final issue is the nature of our inquiry. Given the holistic approach we took, to reduce the burden of survey participation we limited the number of questions we asked in any one domain. In some cases, our findings point to avenues where deeper inquiries would be fruitful rather than providing comprehensive exploration of a given issue. This is a problem for many studies and is one of the reasons ongoing analysis of the multitude of potential challenges and interventions continues to be worthwhile.

The current work also revealed some areas where our baseline survey could be improved. The passage of time is a factor to consider, as well, because as the survey was fielded and results were compiled, the Air Force was not sitting still but was instead engaged in its own quality improvement efforts. Thus, some changes to the second wave of the survey include items asking about other services that, while sometimes offered by the Air Force informally, have been codified since the fielding of the baseline survey (e.g., the role of the Family Liaison Officer). We also included items to increase the breadth of the initial program satisfaction and usage items and to help interpret them. We included items to assess whether reintegration services are helpful. In addition to items that assess satisfaction, we added items that assess the desired call frequency of the AFW2 program. Further, our baseline instrument was limited in that it did not indicate *where* all barriers to mental health care were encountered, and we have modified the survey to include items directly querying in which system(s) of care barriers were met for the barriers seen as the top three most important by each airman. Given the concerns regarding work skills and the educational benefits provided to airmen, we were also able to include an additional item asking about educational pursuits.[2] Finally, in the course of examining our results, we realized that limiting our survey of employment barriers to only those seeking work or those who considered themselves to be disabled excluded consideration of the very real challenges faced by those airmen who had found other employment or who were still with the Air Force. Given the length of the initial baseline survey, making these changes did require cuts to other content domains; however, we feel that the holistic intent and ultimate usefulness of the survey for policymakers will have been retained.

As a final caveat, we should note that since our study was undertaken, the Air Force Wounded Warrior and Air Force Recovery Care Coordinator programs may have modified some of their plans and processes as part of their efforts to expand outreach and improve their processes. We have indicated such changes when they have been brought to our attention, but others may have occurred that are not described here.

---

[2] We thank the reviewer who suggested this addition.

Mental Health

A substantial proportion of airmen who screened positive for current mental health disorders reported encountering barriers to mental health treatment at some point during the past year. Some of the most commonly reported barriers included the belief that available mental health treatments were not very good, concerns about the side effects of psychotropic medication, and concerns about confidentiality and the potentially adverse effects that seeking treatment could have on the level of respect received from one's colleagues and on one's career. Our recommendations are designed to deal with these reported barriers to accessing mental health services. To overcome these barriers to mental health treatment, we recommend that the Air Force (and other related systems of care) take the following actions to increase airmen's receipt of high-quality mental health treatment:

- Inform airmen about the quality of care available to them.
- Evaluate, emphasize, and enhance confidential treatment options.

Next we describe in greater detail how each recommendation might be implemented by the Air Force, including the nonmedical case managers in the AFW2 program and the AFRCC program, and the systems of care that serve wounded, ill, and injured airmen, and offer other relevant suggestions.

Inform Airmen About the Quality of Care Available to Them

Nearly half of airmen with unmet mental health treatment needs perceive that the mental health treatments available to them are not very good. Certainly, as noted earlier, mental health treatments that rest on a substantive evidence base are available for many of the mental health challenges facing these airmen, including PTSD and MDD. Moreover, the Departments of Defense and Veterans Affairs have jointly promulgated evidence-based treatment guidelines for these and other conditions that may be consequences of current conflicts (see, e.g., The Management of Post-Traumatic Stress Working Group, 2010). Given these treatment guidelines, such evidence-based treatments should be easily accessible within both the military and veteran health care systems.

Although the DoD/VA treatment guidelines are evidence-based, concerns have been raised about the extent to which evidence-based treatments are actually provided to patients who receive treatment in the DoD and the VA (Burnam et al., 2008; IOM, 2012; Peterson et al., 2011; Rosen et al., 2004). Even the VA, whose mental health care has been shown to outperform that provided in civilian settings, has demonstrated marked variation in quality of care across its VISNs (Watkins et al., 2011), indicating room for improvement. There are also known concerns regarding the quality of care available on the civilian market (IOM, 2005; President's New Freedom Commission on Mental

Health, 2003; Burnam et al., 2008), which for some of these airmen may represent both the primary source of treatment and one of the more desired sources.

Notwithstanding these findings, concerns about the quality of care provided to patients are at least partly attributable to insufficient assessment, tracking, and reporting of the implementation of evidence-based treatments in practice across health care systems, including the VA, DoD, TRICARE, and civilian settings (Burnam et al., 2008; IOM, 2012). Calls for increased attention to the measurement of the quality of care in the DoD and VA (Burnam et al., 2008) and TRICARE (IOM, 2010) have been issued. Some efforts have been reported to be under way to improve the measurement and tracking of the implementation of evidence-based care in the VA;[3] it is unclear if the DoD has similar plans (IOM, 2012). As of the time of this writing, this quality assessment information is not public. Nevertheless, much remains to be done across health care systems (VA, DoD, TRICARE, and civilian settings) to improve the measurement of quality of care. Thus, to convince airmen of the effectiveness of available treatments, it will be necessary to continue to *collect and publicize data on the quality of care that is implemented*. Many challenges accompany measurement of the quality of care provided to patients (Peterson et al., 2011; Ruzek and Rosen; Shafran et al., 2009). However, as ongoing measurement of the quality of care provided is critical to ensuring that evidence-based treatments adhere to the treatment protocol and are therefore likely to exert beneficial influences on mental health (Burnam et al., 2008), such efforts serve a dual purpose.

Until a more complete picture of the quality of care provided across health care settings is available, airmen should be informed about the care available to them based on what is currently known about the quality of care provided in different health care settings, i.e., where they are most likely to receive high-quality care. Specifically, retired airmen, reservists, and guardsmen may be advised to seek care at the VA rather than a civilian setting,[4] given that the extant research suggests that, on average, airmen are likely to receive higher-quality care in the VA than in a civilian setting (Watkins et al., 2011).

---

[3] At the time of the publication of the IOM (2012) report, there was no capability to track the provision of evidence-based treatments in the VA centralized databases. However, it was reported that the VHA was creating progress note templates for two evidence-based types of psychotherapy for PTSD, cognitive-processing therapy (CPT) and prolonged exposure (PE), to permit recording of the care provided in a way that will permit aggregation of the data collected (Desai, 2011, as cited in IOM, 2012).

[4] Although only the VA can determine eligibility of each case for VHA care, most wounded airmen who are retired would likely be eligible for VHA care based on the following eligibility criteria: (1) All OEF/OIF veterans are eligible for VHA care for five years after service separation, and (2) All veterans who have a service-connected disability are eligible for VHA care. Since nearly all of the retirees in our sample deployed as part of OEF/OIF and all are medically retired (i.e., likely would receive an SC disability rating from VA), it follows that most of them would likely be eligible for VHA care.

To facilitate airmen's receipt of high-quality care in any setting in which they seek or receive treatment, we also recommend *educating airmen about the characteristics of evidence-based treatments so that they will be prepared to identify providers of high-quality care and advocate for their receipt of it* (see, e.g., Pickett et al., 2012). For example, airmen could be informed about the importance of seeking treatment that research has shown to benefit their condition (i.e., evidence-based treatment) and told about the types of treatment whose efficacy has empirical support (e.g., cognitive processing therapy and prolonged exposure are types of evidence-based psychotherapy for PTSD). Airmen could also be coached in the types of questions to ask prospective mental health care providers to gauge their likelihood of delivering high-quality care, such as questions about their training as a clinician, how they make decisions about what type of treatment to provide their patients (are the decisions based on research?), how and whether they keep abreast of the latest developments in mental health care and research, and the manuals that they use to inform their treatment approach (see Brown, 2013).

Another area in which airmen may benefit from education and information about mental health treatment is in understanding of psychotropic medication and its side effects. In our research, although the great majority of airmen who needed mental health treatment reported having received medication for mental health problems at some point in the past year, many airmen reported concerns regarding medication side effects (45 percent of those who reported unmet mental health needs). There is variability in the effects that different medications administered for the same condition have on a given individual and variability in response (including level of concern regarding a given side effect) to the same medication across individuals with the same condition (see Kravitz, Duan, and Braslow, 2004). A relevant example of these issues would be that an individual with MDD may respond differently to various SSRIs that are commonly prescribed for MDD, and the same SSRI can have diverse effects on different individuals being treated for MDD. Thus, finding the medication that strikes the best balance between maximizing symptom relief and minimizing side effects can be a process of trial-and-error for the prescribing physician and the patient (see also Chewning and Sleath's 1996 discussion of the client-centered approach in medication management; Deegan and Drake, 2006). Given these issues, *airmen should be encouraged to raise their concerns about side effects with the prescribing provider* so that the provider can recommend a medication that will minimize side effects of greatest concern to the airmen. Moreover, given the availability of multiple evidence-based psychotropic medications for a given condition such as PTSD or MDD, airmen should be apprised that if one type of medication produces adverse side effects, their providers will work with them to find a medication that best meets their needs. Ideally, such information would be readily available in treatment waiting rooms, but dissemination through discussions with providers and with medical and nonmedical case managers may also be appropriate.

Alternatively, airmen who would forgo mental health treatment altogether because of concerns about the side effects of psychotropic medication should be *encouraged to consider seeking evidence-based psychotherapy without medication.* Although the DoD/VA guidelines for treatment of PTSD and depression recommend both medication and psychotherapy as the optimal treatment approach, there are types of psychotherapy that have demonstrated efficacy in the treatment of PTSD (trauma-focused CBT such as PE; IOM, 2012) and depression (CBT, interpersonal therapy; Cascalenda et al., 2002; Mello et al., 2005) in the absence of medication. Airmen who are opposed to receiving pharmacotherapy for mental health conditions would most likely be better served by receiving evidence-based psychotherapy alone than receiving no mental health treatment at all.

Emphasize and Enhance Confidential Treatment Options

Another barrier to mental health treatment commonly reported by airmen pertained to concerns regarding treatment confidentiality. Our findings show that approximately half of respondents with unmet treatment needs reported one or more of the following: concerns about confidentiality and concerns that treatment seeking would negatively affect the respect of their colleagues and their career (which, if treatment were confidential, would be mitigated as concerns). Thus, we recommend that the Air Force and related systems of care *emphasize and enhance confidential treatment options for airmen* who would otherwise forgo treatment if it were not confidential.

Stigma is a well-recognized concern in the military health system, and efforts are ongoing to combat the issue. Hoge et al. (2004) noted that concerns regarding stigma were strongest among soldiers and marines with mental health needs, that is, among those who screened positive for PTSD, anxiety, or MDD. Others have shown that symptom reporting is higher in situations where anonymity or confidentiality are assured (Warner et al., 2011), with the implication being that servicemembers had incentives to minimize their symptoms when they would be "visible" to the military health system. More recently, Elbogen et al. (2013) reported that servicemembers who had at least one treatment session—that is, those who were actively seeking help—were more likely to report perceptions of stigma than those not in treatment (see also Olmsted et al., 2011). As they noted, once in treatment, it is difficult to minimize one's mental health problems. Actually seeking treatment may also raise concern about the possible consequences of stigma. Kim et al. (2011) indicated that perceptions regarding confidentiality and stigma were inversely related to treatment seeking among recently deployed servicemembers. Moreover, they found that confidentiality concerns were positively associated with seeking treatment on the civilian market, which also echoes the findings in this analysis. Our findings also indicate that these stigma-related concerns are more acute among those who are not yet retired. Collectively, these findings suggest that confidentiality would greatly benefit those who most acutely need treatment, including those who may already be in the system. This is particularly important for those airmen on active duty.

Some confidential nonmedical counseling options are available to servicemembers. Nonmedical counseling is short-term, solution-focused counseling focused on improving clients' functioning in general life areas such as relationship issues, parenting, decisionmaking, stress management, and grief and loss (IOM, 2014). The two main nonmedical counseling programs sponsored by the DoD are Military OneSource and Military and Family Life Consultant (MFLC). Both services are free and provided by master's- or doctorate-level licensed mental health counselors (Weinick et al., 2011).

To date, the DoD has sponsored two completed studies of these programs. In one study, the use of nonmedical counseling by active-duty servicemembers and their spouses was assessed in the May 2010 Military Family Life Project survey (DMDC, 2011). Military OneSource was the second most commonly used provider of counseling services after TRICARE medical counseling services; more than one-half of survey respondents reported that Military OneSource counseling was "helpful." Another study collected survey data from MFLC program participants to assess satisfaction with counseling received from MFLC (DoD, 2012a). Nearly all survey respondents (98 percent) indicated that the counseling from MFLC helped them to deal more effectively with their problems and that they had received the type of counseling they desired (99 percent). Although these findings are encouraging, they are based solely on cross-sectional survey data on perceived benefits of the programs. The cross-sectional designs of these studies preclude inferences regarding the extent to which these programs actually produce their intended benefits. That is, stronger evidence of the programs' effects on their targeted outcomes (i.e., outcomes evaluations that have an experimental or quasi-experimental design) is needed to know whether these programs actually work as intended and should be promoted. Fortunately, both of these programs are being evaluated as part of a five-year (FY 2013–FY 2017) program evaluation of DoD-wide family support programs (DoD, 2012b). The evaluations of Military OneSource and MFLC will examine the effect on outcomes of face-to-face counseling provided by these programs.

Until stronger evidence of these nonmedical counseling programs' effectiveness is available, we recommend that the Air Force case managers promote use of these programs primarily for wounded airmen whose concerns about the confidentiality of mental health treatment are so great that they would otherwise decline any form of treatment. That is, for airmen who have severe PTSD, depression, and/or other mental health conditions, medical counseling that is explicitly designed to target these conditions would typically be the preferred treatment option. However, given that confidential medical counseling is not available through the DoD, and confidential medical counseling provided by mental health professionals outside of the DoD is not free, free

DoD-sponsored nonmedical counseling services may be the best treatment option available to airmen who are concerned about the confidentiality of treatment.

Another confidential source available to military servicemembers is chaplains; however, they are typically not mental health professionals, and their capabilities in this regard have not been systematically evaluated (Besterman-Dahan et al., 2012; cf. Sloan, Marx, and Keane, 2011). As with Military OneSource and the MFLC program, this avenue is considered nonmedical rather than a confidential source for psychotherapy, which is a clinical service. Sloan, Marx, and Keane describe some initiatives undertaken through the Department of Veterans Affairs that also show promise. Echoing the recommendation of a recently conducted study on DoD suicide prevention programs in which NCOs expressed preference for referring suicidal servicemembers to chaplains over behavioral health care providers (Ramchand et al., 2014), we recommend that chaplains be trained to provide evidence-based nonmedical counseling so that they can serve effectively as a high-quality resource for confidential counseling.

In terms of clinical care, efforts are under way to reduce or eliminate the stigma associated with seeking mental health treatment (see, e.g., the description of programs in Weinick et al., 2011), and some limited work suggests that mental health treatment-seeking is unlikely to result in adverse career effect (Christensen and Yaffe, 2012). The Air Force also seeks to *make mental health providers more accessible (and access to them somewhat less visible) by embedding them in primary care clinics* through the Behavioral Health Optimization Program (C. Munsey, 2009). These efforts, too, are important, especially in light of Wong et al.'s (2013) finding that previously deployed active-duty servicemembers are more likely to seek aid from a mental health specialist provider rather than a primary care provider, perhaps owing to a preference for therapy rather than medication. Though the current project was unable to tie perceived barriers with the treatment setting in which they were experienced, future research is planned to make this linkage more definitive and enable further targeted intervention efforts.

Seek Ways to Address Scheduling Difficulties

Concerns regarding stigma issues and confidentiality were not the only ones reported by these injured and ill airmen, however. Nearly one-half of those airmen who reported having desired but not obtained mental health treatment in the past year reported that one of the barriers to care was difficulty scheduling an appointment. Scheduling difficulties have several possible causes, including a shortage of mental health care providers, inflexible clinic hours (e.g., clinics don't offer appointments in the evenings or on weekends), and difficulty navigating the bureaucracy of the medical clinic to reach the point of contact who handles appointment scheduling. Although developing specific options to resolve these issues was not within the scope of our study, efforts should be made to address them. An example of an approach that may be implemented by the Air

Force is *having the nonmedical case managers for both the AFW2 and AFRCC programs help to address scheduling difficulties by assisting airmen in calling the clinic to schedule an appointment.* This suggestion is based on the assumption that difficulty navigating bureaucracy is one of the causes of appointment scheduling difficulties and that the case managers in both of these programs will be able to navigate the bureaucracy effectively at least some of the time. As these assumptions have not been tested, we offer this as a suggestion and acknowledge that it may not be an effective remedy for appointment scheduling difficulties.

Scheduling difficulty may also in part result from ongoing difficulties both the services and the VA have experienced with regard to maintaining sufficient staffing to meet the mental health service demand. In 2007, the Department of Defense Task Force on Mental Health reported insufficient resources to meet demand; more recently the IOM (2012) indicated that evidence regarding whether the DoD and the VA have been able to sufficiently mitigate this shortfall is inadequate. Wells et al. (2011; see also IOM, 2012) summarized a number of initiatives undertaken by the branches of service and the VA to meet the ongoing and likely future demand for mental health services, including efforts at prevention and innovative service provision. They noted that the National Institute of Mental Health (NIMH) is also fully engaged in research efforts to aid the cause. We recommend additional research to shed light on the causes of appointment scheduling difficulties so that more targeted solutions to this problem can be developed.

Employment

Employment is another realm in which nonmedical case managers within the Air Force assist in recovery and reintegration. Many of our respondents indicated that they are currently employed at least part time. However, our results suggest that the unemployment rate is somewhat elevated. Despite the expectation that reported unemployment would typically be higher for those immediately or recently leaving service, this finding still warrants attention and monitoring.

Those working at least part time indicated that they felt their average performance over the past month was somewhat above the typical worker's performance. This is a self-rating of performance; given the study situation, peer or superior evaluations are untenable and, moreover, all rating sources have their own biases (see Newman et al., 2003, for a comprehensive review of that literature). However, we conclude that those airmen who are currently employed feel that they are reasonable contributors to the workforce.[5] The average estimate for absenteeism was that airmen lost between five and

---

[5] In evaluating this average perceived performance rating, the reader should keep in mind the high proportion of our sample who screened positive for depression—and the research finding that depressed

six hours of work over a seven-day period. That is, on average they worked less than their employers expected them to work over that period of time, although there was wide variation in this measure, and other employees indicated that they worked many more hours than anticipated (keep in mind, also, that employers could anticipate more than 40 hours a week).

For those who indicated they were unemployed and looking for work or unemployed because of their disability, we asked about perceived barriers to employment and found that many felt that their disability was a barrier. Given that the majority of respondents who reported that they *were disabled* and not working, concerns regarding disability status are rational and not necessarily an avenue for intervention. However, self-efficacy training is beneficial for others who are having difficulties finding employment (Wanberg, 2012), and specific career counseling can help inform airmen of what options are open to individuals with regard to reasonable accommodations at work. Therefore, these are possible approaches for intervention even when work does not seem an attainable goal initially. As part of the employment counseling assistance already provided through AFW2, case managers may make recommendations for such services and monitor the results to determine if this specific type of assistance is of value for this population.

Offered Employment Assistance Should Focus on Individual Skill Sets and Their Translation to New Contexts

Aside from disability, other reported barriers are potentially more amenable avenues for intervention. For example, some respondents felt concern regarding their qualifications, in particular that their deployments put them behind their civilian counterparts (42 percent), or they reported a general lack of confidence (42 percent). The literature suggests that attention to individual skill sets and their presentation on resumes and in interviews, as well as individual preferences, pays dividends in the forms of employment, lasting employment, and satisfaction (Drake, Bond, and Becker, 2012; Resnick, Rosenheck, and Drebing, 2006; Wanberg, 2012). Moreover, there are many employment aid offerings, and some of the most densely resourced are those provided for wounded, ill, and injured warriors (GAO, 2012, noted 19 different programs in FY 2010). Thus, we do not recommend additional programs, but rather suggest that the *employment assistance offered to airmen focus on individual skill sets and their translation to new contexts*. Specifically, there is a plethora of training options available for veterans generally, and those with combat injuries in particular. Thus, AFW2 assistance can be

---

individuals have more accurate self-perceptions (see DiNisi and Sonesh, 2011, for a discussion of these issues).

used to point these airmen to programs that offer credentialing for experience gained during service, or provide the training and education necessary to leverage such experience and interests.

Reserve Component Members Need Continuing Attention

Across the domains examined, the Reserve and Guard personnel evidenced a higher level of stressors that may strain personal resources to deal with further challenges. They indicated more severe symptoms of mental health disorders and subsequently met screening criteria for mental health diagnoses at a higher rate than active component active-duty airmen. In terms of experienced barriers to care, they were more likely to indicate that they were unsure of where to go to get help. On the positive side, they were also more likely to be in treatment and receiving both medication and therapy. Within the domain of employment, Reserve and Guard personnel who indicated that they were employed at least part time also indicated that their productivity was lower than did our other duty status groups. Wells et al. (2011) summarized other work that suggests that the Reserve and Guard personnel may experience increased vulnerability to deployment-related stressors. These findings, in tandem with the current project findings, suggest continued attention to the needs of the reserve components will be necessary to make sure the care they receive meets their needs.

Conclusion

The process of recovery and reintegration is likely to be lengthy for wounded airmen. A long-term approach is needed to gauge the effectiveness of the many interventions and conditions that affect this process. Thus, we suggest ongoing program evaluation. Many studies have examined various aspects of the problem, but much remains to be done. Moreover, as no one analysis can encompass the complexities that inhere in real life, it is appropriate to leverage quality research from multiple avenues. The Air Force, by means of this and other research, is starting to compile the necessary information. Our data are cross-sectional in nature. We therefore present a snapshot of wounded airmen's well-being on a holistic set of indicators in the fall of 2011. Our findings reveal that enrollees in the Air Force Wounded Warrior program are facing a variety of reintegration challenges. These are likely to remain pressing for some time to come; the Air Force and others must continue to provide support through this process. In a time of declining resources, research can help determine the most effective means to do so.

A. Detailed Measures Information

Relationships and Social Support

Respondents were asked to indicate their current relationship status. Response options included married and living together, married and living separately by choice, married and living separately due to separate military assignments, living together as married, dating exclusively, and no current exclusive relationship. An indicator for marital status was created such that individuals were considered married if they endorsed either of the options "married and living together" or "married and living separately due to separate military assignments," and individuals who endorsed any other relationship status were considered not married.[1]

Respondents were also asked how many dependents they had: "How many children do you have by birth or adoption who depend on you for more than half of their financial support?" For every dependent, respondents were asked the dependent's age and whether or not he or she lived with the respondent.

Respondents also reported their household structure: "Who is living with you for more than half the time?" Response options included spouse or domestic partner, children, parent(s)/parent(s)-in-law, sibling(s)/sibling(s)-in-law, other relatives, and others not related to the respondent.

Respondents were also asked to nominate their primary supporter, i.e., the person "who most often helps you deal with problems that come up." Response options included spouse or domestic partner, boyfriend or girlfriend, child, parent/parent-in-law, brother/brother-in-law or sister/sister-in-law, other relative, friend, or not applicable (don't share problems with anyone).

Respondents rated their satisfaction with their marriage if they were married and living together, married and living separately by choice, or married and living separately due to separate military assignments. Respondents who were not in any of these categories were instead asked to rate their satisfaction with their relationship with their primary supporter. Satisfaction was assessed with a single item: Taking things all

---

[1] We considered including respondents in the category "married and living separately by choice" in the "married" category of the marital status indicator because they are technically married, at least according to the legal definition. However, because these individuals are separated by choice, we believed that they may be categorically different from individuals who are married and not making motions to end their marriage. Thus, we opted to exclude them from the "married" category.

together, how satisfied are you with ("your marriage" if respondent was married; "the relationship you have with the person who most often helps you deal with problems" if respondent was not married)? Response options ranged from very satisfied (1) to very dissatisfied (5). Responses were recoded so that higher scores indicate higher levels of relationship satisfaction.

Respondents were also asked about their perceptions of the social support available to them from different people in their lives. Two subscales from the Social Provisions Scale (Cutrona and Russell, 1987) were used to assess two different dimensions of social support: (1) Reliable Alliance, which refers to the availability of instrumental support (e.g., people to depend on in an emergency), and (2) Attachment, which refers to the availability of emotional support from and intimacy with other people. Sample items from the Reliable Alliance subscale include: "There are people I can depend on to help me if I really need it," and "If something went wrong, no one would come to my assistance." Sample items from the Attachment subscale include "I feel that I do not have close personal relationships with other people," and "I have close relationships that provide me with a sense of emotional security and well-being." Past research has demonstrated the reliability, convergent validity, and divergent validity of the SPS (Cutrona and Russell, 1987). Each subscale consists of four items, each of which is rated on a Likert scale with response options ranging from strongly disagree (1) to strongly agree (4). Possible scores on the Reliable Alliance and Attachment subscales range from 4 to 16. Subscale items are scored and aggregated so that higher subscale scores connote higher levels of perceived social support. Internal consistency reliability estimates for both of these subscales were very high in the current analysis (Reliable Alliance: Cronbach's alpha = 0.87; Attachment: Cronbach's alpha = 0.81).

TBI Screening

We screened for the occurrence of a TBI during deployment or deployment-related activities with the Brief Traumatic Brain Injury Scale (BTBIS), a measure that has been used by the military with servicemembers returning from OEF/OIF (Schwab et al., 2007). Respondents screened positive for the occurrence of a TBI if they endorsed any injury during deployment from a fragment, bullet, vehicular accident, fall, explosion (e.g., IED), or something else and reported having experienced an alteration in consciousness right after the injury, such as being dazed, confused, or "seeing stars"; not remembering the injury; or having a loss of consciousness (LOC) for any length of time (Schwab et al., 2005). Response options for LOC were broken down into three different intervals of time: LOC for less than one minute, between one and 20 minutes, and greater than 20 minutes.

PTSD Screening

The PTSD Checklist (PCL; Weathers et al., 1993), an instrument that contains 17 symptom items keyed directly to the Diagnostic and Statistical Manual of Mental Disorders, Fourth Edition (DSM-IV; American Psychiatric Association, 1994), was used to screen for PTSD. Respondents indicated the extent to which they had been bothered by each symptom in the past 30 days on a scale with response options ranging from 1 (not at all) to 5 (extremely). The PCL has been used to study post-traumatic distress in various military samples (e.g., Grieger et al., 2006) and is commonly used to screen for PTSD in both the Department of Defense (DoD) and the Veterans Health Administration (VHA).

Respondents were classified as screening positive for PTSD in accordance with guidelines offered by Weathers et al. (1993). Symptoms were counted as present if respondents indicated that they had been at least "moderately (3)" bothered by the symptom. Based on the DSM-IV definition, also known as the cluster scoring method, respondents were classified as screening positive or negative for PTSD. This scoring has been shown to have high sensitivity and specificity, 1.00 and 0.92, respectively (see Brewin, 2005, for a review of different scoring methods).

MDD Screening

The Patient Health Questionnaire-8 (PHQ-8; Kroenke, Spitzer, and Williams, 2001; Lowe, Kroenke, et al., 2004) was used to screen for MDD. The PHQ-8 assesses all of the criteria on which a DSM-IV diagnosis of MDD is based except for suicidal ideation. Responses to the PHQ-8 are provided with respect to the frequency with which symptoms were experienced in the past two weeks on a four-point (0–3) scale. The PHQ-8 is well validated and widely used as a brief screening measure in civilian settings (e.g., Lowe, Spitzer, et al., 2004) and in the DoD and VA. Respondents were classified as screening positive for MDD if they had a total score of 10 or above on the PHQ-8, following the recommended cut-point (Kroenke, Spitzer, and Williams, 2001). This cut-point yields a sensitivity of 0.99 and a specificity of 0.92, which is slightly more specific than the PHQ-9 (Kroenke et al., 2001).

Alcohol Consumption and Misuse

We screened for alcohol misuse with the Alcohol Use Disorders Identification Test—Consumption (AUDIT-C; Bush, Kivlahan, McDonell, Fihn, and Bradley, 1998). The AUDIT-C has been validated in past research as a screener for identification of individuals with heavy drinking and/or active alcohol abuse or dependence in past research (Bush et al., 1998). This scale consists of three items that assess quantity and frequency of typical and heavy drinking. Participants answer each item on a 0–4 scale, and composite scores are computed by summing item scores. In the current research, alcohol misuse was defined by a score of 4 or higher in males and a score of 3 or higher in females, consistent with the cutoffs used by the VHA (Achtmeyer and Bradley, 2011). In past research, this cutoff for males has been shown to have a sensitivity of 0.86 and a specificity of 0.72 in VA outpatients and a sensitivity of 0.86 and specificity of 0.89 in non-VA outpatients (Achtmeyer and Bradley, 2011). This cutoff in females has been shown to have a sensitivity of 0.66 and specificity of 0.94 in VA outpatients and a sensitivity of 0.73 and specificity of 0.91 in non-VA outpatients (Achtmeyer and Bradley, 2011).

Illicit Drug Use

Respondents' use of illicit substances during the previous 12 months was assessed with the following question, "In the past 12 months have you used any _____?" with respect to three different categories of illicit substances: (1) marijuana, (2) other illegal drugs, including cocaine, opium, amphetamines, or Ecstasy, and (3) any prescription medication that was not prescribed for the respondent by a doctor or was used in a way other than as prescribed.

Mental Health Services Utilization and Preferences

Utilization of any type of mental health services in the previous year was assessed with a single question: "In the past 12 months have you received any of the following types of treatment for stress, emotional, alcohol, drug, or family problems?" Response options included medication prescribed by a mental health care provider, some type of counseling or talk therapy provided by a mental health specialist, and some other treatment. Respondents who endorsed any of these response options were considered to have received some sort of mental health treatment in the past year. For every type of treatment the respondent reported having received, the respondent was asked to indicate all of the settings in which he or she had received that type of treatment. Response options included military treatment facility, VA facility, and civilian facility.

Respondents were also asked to indicate their preferred type of provider if cost were not an issue: "If you wanted to get mental health care and could go to any type of provider free of charge, would you go to…" Response options were mutually exclusive (i.e., the respondent could choose only one option) and included military treatment facility, VA facility, civilian facility, and none of these. Preferences for type of treatment were also assessed: "If you wanted to get mental health care and could afford any of the following types of treatment, which one of the following treatments would you choose?" The mutually exclusive response options included medication prescribed by a health care provider, some type of counseling or talk therapy provided by a mental health specialist, and neither.

Unmet Need for Mental Health Services and Barriers to Care

To assess unmet need for mental health services during the previous year, we asked respondents a single question: "In the past 12 months was there ever a time when you wanted to get professional help for a mental health, stress, family or alcohol problem but did not?" Respondents who answered "yes" to this question were then read a list of 12 concerns and asked to select those that had kept them from getting help when they needed it. Respondents who answered "no" were read the same list of concerns and asked to indicate which concerns would make it difficult for them to get help in the future if they needed it. The concerns on the list were drawn from previous studies of mental health treatment barriers conducted in military samples (Schell and Marshall, 2008; Vaughan et al., 2011). Original sources of the barriers include the National Comorbidity Survey Replication (NCS-R) (e.g., Kessler et al., 2005) and the Hoge et al. (2004) study of barriers to care in the military. The list comprises three broad classes of barriers to care: logistical barriers (e.g., "difficulty scheduling an appointment"), institutional and cultural barriers ("concerns about harm being done to your career"), and beliefs and preferences for treatment (e.g., "believing that the mental health treatments available to you are not very good").

Physical Health

The Medical Outcomes Study Short Form 36 General Health Survey (SF-36; Ware, Snow, Kosinski, and Gandek, 1993) subscales of general health and role limitations due to physical health were used to assess respondents' physical health. General health was self-reported on a scale that ranged from 1 (excellent) to 5 (poor). Role limitations due to physical health were assessed with four items asking the respondent about the occurrence of four problems with "work or other regular daily activities as a result of your physical health" during the past four weeks. Both subscales were scored in accordance with the recommendations of Hays, Sherbourne, and Mazel (1993). Subscale scores range from 0 to 100, with higher scores indicating better health. The reliability and validity of the SF-36 have been extensively documented in past research (Brazier et al., 1992; Buchwald et al., 1996; Stansfeld, Roberts, and Foot, 1997; Ware et al., 1993).

Employment Status

Respondents were asked to select their current employment status from a list that included the following options: "working full time," "working part time," "unemployed and looking for work," "disabled and not working," "full-time student," "part-time student," "homemaker," "retired," and "not employed, not looking for work." Employment status was then defined two ways. One method used the entire sample as the denominator and divided the sample into mutually exclusive categories of current employment status for descriptive purposes. The other method used the denominator defined in the U3 measure of unemployment used by the Bureau of Labor Statistics (BLS, 2010). This denominator is restricted to the civilian workforce, defined as individuals who are currently employed either part or full time and those who are unemployed and looking for work. The numerator was the number of individuals who reported that they were unemployed and looking for work.

Job Performance and Satisfaction

The absenteeism and presenteeism questions from the World Health Organization Health and Work Performance Questionnaire (WHO HPQ; Kessler et al., 2003) were used to assess absenteeism and presenteeism in respondents who were employed part or full time. Absolute absenteeism was computed based on respondents' self-reports of the total number of hours that they had worked in the past seven days and the number of hours that their employers expected them to work in a typical seven-day week. Both of these numbers were multiplied by four to convert estimates for the past week to a month, and then the estimated number of hours that the respondent had worked in the past month was subtracted from the estimated number of hours that the respondent's employer expected him or her to work during the past month. Positive values indicate hours of work lost, with higher positive values indicating more hours of work lost, i.e., greater absenteeism. A value of zero indicates no hours of work lost (i.e., the number of hours actually worked was equal to the number of hours of work expected by the employer), and negative values indicate that the respondent worked more than his or her employer expects. The maximum and minimum values allowed on each of these absenteeism questions are 97 and zero, respectively, and thus the range of possible scores is -388 to 388.

Absolute presenteeism was computed based on a question asking individuals to "rate your overall job performance on the days you worked during the past four weeks (28 days)" on a scale that ranged from 0 (worst performance) to 10 (top performance). Their self-rating was then multiplied by 100 to represent their presenteeism score as a percentage. Absolute presenteeism scores therefore range from 0 to 100, with higher scores indicating higher self-perceived job performance.

Job satisfaction was assessed with a single question: "How satisfied are you with your job in general?" Response options ranged from 1 (very dissatisfied) to 5 (very satisfied).

This single-item measure of job satisfaction has been validated in past research (Scarpello and Campbell, 1983; Weiss et al., 1967).

Work Involvement

Respondents were also asked questions about their work involvement. This construct pertains to the centrality of work to one's life, as opposed to work simply being a way to earn money. Based on a measure developed by Warr et al. (1979), six questions about work involvement were asked. Sample items include "Having a job is very important to me," and "I would soon get very bored if I had no work to do." Response options for each item ranged from disagree a lot (1) to agree a lot (5). Internal consistency reliability for this set of items was good in the current sample (Cronbach's alpha = 0.83). Items were summed to obtain a composite scale score, with higher scores indicating greater perceived centrality of work to one's life.

Vocational Rehabilitation Services Utilization

Respondents were asked to indicate whether they had received vocational rehabilitation services from any of the following settings: military program, a VA program, or another program.

Barriers to Employment

Respondents whose current employment status was "disabled and not working" or "unemployed and looking for work" were asked to indicate which of 16 potential barriers to employment "make it difficult for you to obtain employment." Barriers assessed in our research were drawn from another survey of wounded warriors (data not publicly releasable). Barriers fell roughly into four major categories: disability-related barriers (e.g., "no one will hire me because of my injury or disability"); concerns about qualifications, skills, or abilities needed for the civilian labor market (e.g., "I lack confidence in myself and my abilities"); disincentives to obtain employment (e.g., "would lose financial benefits"); and other (e.g., "do not know about available jobs").

Financial Strain

Financial strain was assessed with two main measures. One indicator of financial strain was the categorization of veterans as above or below the federal poverty guidelines set by the U.S. Department of Health and Human Service for 2010 (DHHS, 2010). This categorization is derived from the respondent's best estimate of his or her household's total annual income from all sources before taxes in 2010 and the number of people in their household supported by their total household income.

The other measure of financial strain consisted of three items designed to assess respondents' self-perceived financial difficulties (Vinokur and Caplan, 1987). Respondents indicated how difficult it was to live on their household income at the present time on a scale that ranged from 1 (not at all difficult) to 5 (extremely difficult or impossible). Respondents also answered two questions about the extent to which they expected to experience, over the next two months, financial adversity such as not having a home or enough food or medical care and having to reduce their lifestyle to the bare necessities. Both of these questions were rated on a scale that ranged from 1 (not at all) to 5 (a great deal). Internal consistency reliability for this scale was good in the current sample (Cronbach's alpha = 0.80). Responses to these three questions were averaged to obtain a composite scale score for financial strain.

Housing Stability

We developed several indicators related to past and current housing situations and stability. In the absence of well-validated measures of the constructs of interest, we solicited input from experts in homelessness (Joan Tucker and Paul Koegel) to inform the development of our indicators. In general, our location items were phrased such that they could be comparable to the conceptualization of homelessness embodied by the McKinney-Vento Homelessness Act.

First, we assessed lifetime history of homelessness by asking airmen whether they had ever spent the night in one of the following locations: a transitional shelter or program; a homeless shelter; in a chapel or church (but not in a bed); an all-night theater or other indoor public place; an abandoned building; a car or vehicle; or the street or other outdoor place. Airmen who endorsed any of these options were considered to have a lifetime history of homelessness; Airmen who did not endorse any of these options were skipped out of the rest of this section of the survey. We then asked airmen about the first and last times they had spent the night in any of the locations that they endorsed in the previous question and used this information to develop indicators of whether they had been homeless for a night since their most recent return from deployment and whether their first time being homeless had occurred since their most recent return from deployment. We also assessed the duration of time that respondents had lived at their current place of residence.

We also asked some more in-depth questions to gauge the stability of respondents' housing situations over the previous six months. Respondents were given a list of different settings in which they might have lived during the previous six months and asked to indicate where they had lived during the previous six months. Settings on the list included the following: their own home; a partner's home; the home of a family member; the home of a friend; a self-paid hotel or motel room; a partner-paid hotel or motel room; a family or friend paid hotel or motel room; a hotel or motel room paid for with a voucher; a boarding, transition or halfway house; a residential alcohol or drug detox program; a psychiatric or drug treatment inpatient facility; a hospital, a jail or prison; a shelter or other program; a mission or shelter; a church or chapel; an all-night theater or similar; an abandoned building; a vehicle; or the street. We classified the following settings as indicative of homelessness in the previous six months: a hotel or motel room paid for with a voucher; a boarding, transition, or halfway house; a mission or shelter; a church or chapel; an all-night theater or similar location; an abandoned building; a vehicle; or the street. Airmen who selected a setting indicative of homelessness were asked how long they had spent there. We classified the following settings as potentially at-risk for homelessness: the home of family or friends; a hotel room paid for by themselves, a partner, or family or friends; residential alcohol or drug detox; a psychiatric hospital or drug treatment facility; and hospital. Respondents who indicated having lived in an apartment or home of their own or a partner's home, apartment, or room were considered not to have been homeless in the past six months. Respondents were also asked to select their current housing situation from the list and were classified as currently homeless or at-risk for homelessness using the same definitions described above.

In addition to applying our objective definitions of homelessness to characterize respondents' living situations, we asked respondents to indicate whether they considered themselves to have been homeless at any time during the previous six months to gauge their self-perception of their housing situation. Finally, we asked respondents who did not currently live in their own or their partner's home to indicate the main reason they did not currently live in their own or their partner's home. Reasons on the list included the following: saving money for my own place; hiding from creditors; cannot afford it; house foreclosed on; enjoy staying with friends/family; left housing due to relationship difficulties with living companions; hard to find quality housing; do not feel it is necessary to live in an apartment or home that you and/or your partner own or rent.

Perceived Helpfulness of Assistance and Services

Respondents were asked to indicate whether each of ten different types of assistance and services would be useful to them, regardless of whether they had ever received it. The types of assistance and services assessed included medical care, financial aid for education, job training, housing assistance or loans, transitional housing, general information (e.g., about rules or policies, or about what's available and how to access it), an advocate (i.e., someone to try to get help for the respondent), help connecting with others on a personal level, a helping hand (e.g., loans, donations, services to help out with some of your responsibilities), and activities (e.g., for fitness, recreation, stress relief, family bonding). Some of these items were drawn from a list of desired types of assistance and services that was used in a previous study of OEF/OIF veterans (Vaughan et al., 2011), and others were created specifically for our project.

Air Force Wounded Warrior Program Utilization and Perceptions

All respondents were asked whether they had had contact with an AFW2 representative. Respondents who answered this question affirmatively were then asked whether this contact was initiated by them (the respondent) or the AFW2 representative and to indicate which of seven types of AFW2 services they had received. Types of AFW2 services assessed included referrals to other services, help or advice for filling out paperwork, advice for life matters, advice for dealing with red tape, whether AFW2 had someone contact the respondent to give him/her assistance, regular supportive calls, and some other help or service.

Respondents who reported having received at least one type of AFW2 service were then asked to indicate whether they agreed or disagreed with several statements designed to assess their perceptions of the services provided by the AFW2 program. Respondents indicated their agreement or disagreement with the following statements: (1) the case managers give me good information on what resources are available to me, (2) the services available through AFW2 case managers can't really help me deal with any issues caused during my Air Force service, (3) I would like for the AFW2 case managers to contact me more often, (4) AFW2 case managers are available and ready to help me if I wanted to contact them, and (5) overall, I am satisfied with the services provided by the AFW2 program.

Air Force Recovery Care Coordinator Program Utilization and Perceptions

Respondents were asked whether they had received any services from the AFRCC program. Respondents who answered this question affirmatively were then asked which of several types of help or services they had received from a Recovery Care Coordinator: (1) assistance with goal-setting and planning for the future through the development of a Comprehensive Recovery Plan (CRP) or Recovery Care Plan (RCP), (2) referrals to other services and programs for veterans or combat-injured airmen, (3) help accessing services and programs for veterans or combat-injured airmen, (4) advice for life matters, (5) regular supportive calls, (6) follow-up after the development of your Comprehensive Recovery Plan and Recovery Care Plan to help you stay on track to meet your goals, (7) help adjusting to or coping with physical or mental health conditions that you developed during or after your military service, and (8) some other help or service.

Several statements designed to assess respondents' perceptions of various aspects of the AFRCC program and potential barriers to program utilization were then asked. Respondents' agreement with the following statements regarding the AFRCC program was assessed: (1) the RCCs can give me good information on what resources are available to me, (2) they can help me get access to the services and programs that I need, (3) they can't really help me deal with any issues or problems caused during my Air Force service, (4) they are easy to get in touch with if I wanted to contact them, (5) others, such as family members, friends, or coworkers, would think less of me for getting help or services from the AFRCC program, (6) my career would be harmed by getting help or services, (7) the RCCs can help me to achieve my personal goals, (8) overall, I am satisfied with the services provided by the AFRCC program.

B. Survey Instrument

AIR FORCE SERVICE HISTORY[1]

[If this is not the respondent's first survey administration **and** the respondent indicated in a previous administration that he or she was in the category "permanent disability retirement" (option 3) in MS1b, skip out of the section on Air Force Service History.]

MS1ab. Have you been referred to the Medical Evaluation Board?
1. Yes
2. No (skip to MS2)
97. Not sure (skip to MS2)
99. Refused (skip to MS2)

MS1b . Which of the following was the outcome of your Physical Evaluation Board? [READ OPTIONS, RECORD SINGLE RESPONSE]
1. Not applicable - I am going through the Medical Evaluation Board but have not been referred to the PEB
2. Permanent disability retirement
3. Placed on the temporary disability retirement list
4. Other
97. Not sure
99. Refused

[If this is not the respondent's first survey administration, skip MS2 and go to MS3.]
MS2. Did you spend most of your career in the Air Force as officer or enlisted?
1. Officer
2. Enlisted
    99. Refused

MS3. Considering all periods during which you were on active duty together, how many total YEARS did you spend on active duty in the military? ____
(Programmer: Program drop-down menu with response options ranging from 0 to 40 years, 99 Refused)

---

[1] Note: this reflects the web version of the survey.

PROGRAM EVALUATION

Air Force Wounded Warrior Questions

PR1. Have you been in contact with a representative of the Air Force Wounded Warrior program? [Notes: If this is not the respondent's first time completing the survey and the respondent provided a valid response (i.e., response other than "don't know" or "refused") to this question in the previous survey, add to the end of the question "since we last spoke with you in (insert month and year of previous survey administration")?"]

1. Yes (Go to PR1a)

2. No (Go to PR5)

3. I'm not sure what the Air Force Wounded Warrior program is (Go to PR5)

99. REF (Go to PR5)

PR1a. Did the representative of the Air Force Wounded Warrior Program contact you first, or did you contact the Air Force Wounded Warrior Program first?

1. The representative of the Air Force Wounded Warrior Program contacted me first.

2. I contacted a representative of the Air Force Wounded Warrior Program first.

99. REF

PR2. What help or services have you received from the Air Force Wounded Warrior program? [If this is not the respondent's first time completing the survey and the respondent provided a valid response to this question in the previous survey, add to the end of the question "since you last completed this survey in (insert month and year of previous survey administration")?"]

[Programmer: Response options include:]

1. Yes

2. No

99. REF

      a. Referrals to other services

      b. Help or advice for filling out paperwork

      c. Advice for life matters

      d. Advice for dealing with red tape

      e. They had someone contact me to give me assistance

      f. Regular supportive calls

g. Some other help or service

[Programmer: If respondent does not answer "yes" to any of items a-g of PR2, skip to PR4]

PR3. Please indicate whether you agree or disagree with each of the following statements about the Air Force Wounded Warrior program.

Response options include:

1. Agree

2. Disagree

99. REF

> a. The case managers give me good information on what resources are available to me.
>
> b. The services available through Air Force Wounded Warrior case managers can't really help me deal with any issues caused during my Air Force service.
>
> c. I would like for the Air Force Wounded Warrior case managers to contact me more often.
>
> d. Air Force Wounded Warrior case managers are available and ready to help me if I wanted to contact them.
>
> e. Overall, I am satisfied with the services provided by the Air Force Wounded Warrior program.

Ask PR4 only if the respondent answered no/not sure/ref to all of pr2a-g, i.e., they have not received help or services.

PR4. Which of the following kept you from receiving any help or services from the Air Force Wounded Warrior Program? [If this is not the respondent's first time completing the survey and the respondent provided a valid response to this question in the previous survey, add to the end of the question "since (insert month and year of previous survey administration")?"]

Response options include:

1. Yes

2. No

99. REF

a. Not knowing what type of services are provided

b. Thinking that the services provided would not be effective in addressing your problems

c. Difficulty contacting the case managers

d. Concerns that information you shared with would not be kept confidential

e. Concerns that others, such as family members, friends, or co-workers, would think less of you for getting help or services from the Air Force Wounded Warrior program

f. Concerns that your career would be harmed by getting help or services

g. Concerns that getting help would lead to more requirements of you, such as time, money, or paperwork

Air Force Recovery Care Coordinator Program Questions

PR5. Have you received any help or services from an Air Force Recovery Care Coordinator? [If this is not the respondent's first time completing the survey and the respondent provided a valid response to this question in the previous survey, add to the end of the question "since (insert month and year of previous survey administration")?"]

1. Yes (ask PR6)

2. No (skip to PR8)

3. Not sure what the Air Force Recovery Care Coordinator program is (skip to PR8)

4. Does not apply (skip to PR8)

99. REF

PR6. What help or services have you received from an Air Force Recovery Care Coordinator? [If this is not the respondent's first time completing the survey and the respondent provided a valid response to this question in the previous survey, add to the end of the question "since (insert month and year of previous survey administration")?"]

[Programmer: Response options include:]

1. Yes

2. No

99. REF

Have you received…

    a. Assistance with goal-setting and planning for the future through the development of a Comprehensive Recovery Plan (CRP) or Recovery Care Plan (RCP)

    b. Referrals to other services and programs for veterans or combat-injured Airmen

    c. Help accessing services and programs for veterans or combat-injured Airmen

    d. Advice for life matters

e. Regular supportive calls

f. Follow-up after the development of your Comprehensive Recovery Plan and Recovery Care Plan to help you stay on track to meet your goals

g. Help adjusting to or coping with physical or mental health conditions that you developed during or after your military service

h. Some other help or service

PR7. Please indicate whether you agree or disagree with the following statements about the Air Force Recovery Care Coordinator program.

Response options include:

1. Agree

2. Disagree

99. REF

a. The Recovery Care Coordinators (RCCs) can give me good information on what resources are available to me.

b. They can help me get access to the services and programs that I need.

c. They can't really help me deal with any issues or problems caused during my Air Force service.

d. They are easy to get in touch with if I wanted to contact them.

e. Others, such as family members, friends, or co-workers, would think less of me for getting help or services from the Recovery Care Coordinator program

f. My career would be harmed by getting help or services

g. The RCCs can help me to achieve my personal goals.

h. Overall, I am satisfied with the services provided by the Recovery Care Coordinator program.

PR8. Veterans and combat-injured Airmen are eligible for a wide range of possible benefits and services. Which of the following benefits, if any, have you received since your most recent deployment or deployment-related activities? [If this is not the respondent's first time completing the survey and the respondent provided a valid answer to this question in his/her previous survey administration, substitute "since (insert month and year of previous survey administration)" for "since your most recent deployment."]

[Programmer: Response options include:]

1. Yes
2. No
99. REF

Have you received...

1. Medical care at any VA facility
2. Assistance at a VA Vet Center
3. Financial aid for education
4. Disability payments
5. Military retirement pay
6. Housing assistance or loans
7. Transitional housing
8. Reduced costs of health insurance for myself or my family members

PR9. For each of the following types of assistance or services, please select "yes" if it would be helpful to you or "no" if it would not be helpful to you, regardless of whether you've ever used it.

Response options:
1. Yes
2. No
98. DK
99. REF

1. Medical care
2. Financial aid for my education
3. Job training
4. Housing assistance or loans
5. Transitional housing
6. General information: for example, about rules or policies, or about what's available and how to access it
7. An advocate: someone to try to get help for you
8. Help connecting with others on a personal level
9. A helping hand: loans, donations, services to help out with some of your responsibilities
10. Activities: for fitness, recreation, stress relief, family bonding

As a reminder, all of these questions are confidential.
PR10. In addition to health insurance you may have through the VA or Tricare, are you currently covered by any other health insurance? This may include health insurance you purchase directly, that you get through an employer or union, or that you get through a spouse or parent.

1. Yes
2. No
99. Refused

MENTAL HEALTH

The following questions are about things that might have happened while you
were in the military.

Trauma History

You are going to be asked about your reactions to difficult or stressful events that
people sometimes experience or witness during deployment or deployment-
related situations. Some examples of this are being in some type of serious
accident; witnessing an accident that resulted in serious injury or death; being
physically moved or knocked over by an explosion; having a friend who was
seriously wounded or killed; seeing dead or seriously injured non-combatants;
or being forced to have sex when you didn't want to.

TE1. While you were deployed, did you experience or witness any events similar
to those just described during which you felt that you or someone else were
going to die or be killed?
1.Yes (go to TE2)
2.No (go to PCL1)
99. REF (go to PCL1)

TE2. Did you feel intense fear, helplessness, or horror during any of these
events?
1. Yes
2. No
99. REF

PTSD Checklist (PCL)

The following is a list of reactions that Airmen sometimes experience following deployment or in response to other stressful life experiences. Please indicate how much you have been bothered by each problem IN THE PAST 30 DAYS.

PCL1. In the past 30 days how bothered have you been by (insert a-q), not at all, a little bit, moderately, quite a bit, or extremely bothered?
(Response options are)

Not at all	A Little Bit	Moderately	Quite a Bit	Extremely	(vol.) Ref
1	2	3	4	5	99

a. Repeated, disturbing *memories, thoughts, or images* of the stressful experience
b. Repeated, disturbing *dreams* of the stressful experience
c. Suddenly *acting* or *feeling* as if the stressful experience were *happening again* (as if you were re-living it)
d. Feeling *very upset* when *something reminded you* of the stressful experience
e. Having *physical reactions* (like heart pounding, trouble breathing, sweating) when *something reminded you* of the stressful experience
f. Avoiding *thinking about* or *talking about* the stressful experience or avoiding *having feeling*s related to it
g. Avoiding *activities* or *situations* because *they reminded you* of the stressful experience
h. Trouble *remembering important parts* of the stressful experience
i. *Loss of interest* in activities that you used to enjoy
j. Feeling *distant* or *cut-off* from other people
k. Feeling *emotionally numb* or being unable to have loving feelings for those close to you
l. Feeling as if your *futur*e somehow will be *cut short*
m. Trouble *falling* or *staying asleep*
n. Feeling *irritable* or having *angry outbursts*
o. Having *difficulty concentrating*
p. Being *"super alert"* or watchful or on-guard
q. Feeling *jumpy* or easily startled

PCL2. [IF ALL PCL1=1, THEN SKIP TO TBI1.] Were these symptoms due to stressful experiences that occurred during a military deployment or other operation or training?
1.Yes
2.No
99. Refused

Brief Traumatic Brain Injury Scale

[Ask TBI1 and TBI2 only of respondents who are completing the survey for the first time or who provided an invalid response during their first survey administration. If respondent says no or not sure to options 1 through 6 of TBI1, skip TBI2 and proceed to next section.]

TBI1. Did you have any injuries during any deployments or deployment-related activities from any of the following? Please select yes or no for each.

[Programmer; Response options include:]
1.Yes
2.No
99. Refused

       1.Fragment
       2.Bullet
       3.Vehicular (any type of vehicle including airplane)
       4.Fall
       5.Explosion (IED, RPG, land mine, grenade, etc.)
       6. Other

TBI2. Did any injury you received while deployed or during related activities result in any of the following? Please select yes or no for each.
Response options:
1.Yes
2.No
98.DK
99. Refused

       1. Being dazed, confused, or "seeing stars"
       2. Not remembering the injury
       3. Losing consciousness (knocked out) for less than a minute
       4. Losing consciousness for 1-20 min
       5. Losing consciousness for longer than 20 min
       6. Having any symptoms of concussion afterward (such as headache, dizziness, irritability, etc.)
       7. Head injury

Depressive Symptoms (Patient Health Questionnaire-8)

Now you will be asked some questions about your mood, and problems that may have bothered you over the last 2 weeks. Please answer just for the last 2 weeks, even if that period has not been usual for you.

D1.   In the last 2 weeks how often have you been bothered by having little interest or pleasure in doing things:

      1   Not at all,
      2   Several days,
      3   More than half the days, or
      4   Nearly every day
      99 REF

D2.   In the last 2 weeks how often have you been bothered by feeling down, depressed, or hopeless?

      1   Not at all,
      2   Several days,
      3   More than half the days, or
      4   Nearly every day
      99 REF

D3.   In the last 2 weeks how often have you been bothered by trouble falling asleep or staying asleep, or sleeping too much?

      1   Not at all,
      2   Several days,
      3   More than half the days, or
      4   Nearly every day
      99 REF

D4.   In the last 2 weeks how often have you been bothered by feeling tired or having little   energy?

      1   Not at all,
      2   Several days,
      3   More than half the days, or
      4   Nearly every day
      99 REF

D5.   In the last 2 weeks how often have you been bothered by poor appetite or overeating?

1 Not at all,

2 Several days,

3 More than half the days, or

4 Nearly every day

99 REF

D6.   In the last 2 weeks how often have you been bothered by feeling bad about yourself – or   that you are a failure or have let yourself or your family down?

1 Not at all,

2 Several days,

3 More than half the days, or

4 Nearly every day

99 REF

D7.   In the last 2 weeks how often have you been bothered by trouble concentrating on things,   such as reading the newspaper or watching television?

1 Not at all,

2 Several days,

3 More than half the days, or

4 Nearly every day

99 REF

D8.   In the last 2 weeks how often have you been bothered by moving or speaking so slowly that other people could have noticed? Or the opposite – being so fidgety or restless that   you were moving around a lot more than usual?

1 Not at all,

2 Several days,

3 More than half the days, or

4 Nearly every day

99 REF

Alcohol Use

[For all questions in the Alcohol Use section, if this is not the respondent's first time completing the survey, replace the time qualifier "in the past 12 months" with "since (insert month and year of previous survey administration)."]

As a reminder, all of these questions are confidential.

AU1. How often did you have a drink containing alcohol in the past 12 months? Consider a "drink" to be a can or bottle of beer, a glass of wine, a wine cooler, or one cocktail or a shot of hard liquor (like scotch, gin, or vodka).

1. Never (skip to DU1)
2. Monthly or less
3. 2 to 4 times a month
4. 2 to 3 times a week
5. 4 to 5 times a week
6. 6 or more times a week
99. REF

AU2. How many drinks did you have on a typical day when you were drinking in the past 12 months?

1. 0 drinks
2. 1 to 2 drinks
3. 3 to 4 drinks
4. 5 to 6 drinks
5. 7 to 9 drinks
6. 10 or more drinks
99. REF

AU3. How often did you have 6 or more drinks on one occasion in the past 12 months?

1. Never
2. Less than monthly
3. Monthly
4. Weekly
5. Daily or almost daily
99. REF

Drug Use

Again, please remember that all of these questions are confidential.

[For all questions in the Drug Use section, if this is not the respondent's first time completing the survey, replace the time qualifier "in the past 12 months" with "since (insert month and year of previous survey administration)."]

DU1. In the past 12 months have you used any marijuana?

    1. Yes
    2. No
    99. Refused

DU2. In the past 12 months have you used any other illegal drugs, this includes cocaine, opium, amphetamines, or ecstasy?
    1. Yes
    2. No
    99. Refused

DU3. In the past 12 months have you used any prescription medication that was not prescribed for you by a doctor, or used these medications in a way different than prescribed?
    1. Yes
    2. No
    99. Refused

Mental Health Treatment History

MH1. In the last 12 months, have you received any of the following types of treatment for stress, emotional, alcohol, drug, or family problems? For each type of treatment, please select "yes" if you have received it or "no" if you have not. [If this is not the respondent's first time completing the survey, replace "In the last 12 months" with "Since (insert month and year of previous survey administration)".]

Response options include:
    1. Yes
    2. No
    99. REF

    a. Medication prescribed by a health care provider.

b. Some type of counseling or talk therapy provided by a mental health specialist such as a psychiatrist, psychologist, counselor, or social worker;
c. Other

(If respondent answers "yes" to a, b, or c of MH1, ask MH2 for each of these; if respondent answers "no" or "refuse" to a, b, and c of MH1, skip to MH3)

MH2. Where did you (receive medication/participate in therapy/receive other treatment)? For each of the following, please select "yes" if you received (medication/participate in therapy/receive other treatment) there or "no" if you did not.

Response options include:
1. Yes
2. No
99. REF

a. Military health facility
b. VA facility
c. Civilian facility

Unmet Need/Desire for Mental Health Treatment

MH3. In the last 12 months, was there ever a time when you wanted to get professional help for stress, emotional, alcohol, drug, or family problems but did not? [If this is not the respondent's first time completing the survey, replace "In the last 12 months" with "Since (insert month and year of previous survey administration)".]

1. Yes
2. No
99. Refused

Barriers to Mental Health Treatment

MH4. (Use different introductory question for each of the following 2 categories):

1) (Ask this of people who indicated in question MH3 above that they did not want treatment): Even when people need to get help for their emotional or personal problems they may find it difficult to get help. If in the future you wanted help for stress, emotional, alcohol, drug, or family problems, which of the following concerns would get in the way of seeking or receiving treatment for any of these problems? Please select yes or no for each concern listed.

2) (Ask this of people who indicated in question MH3 above that they wanted help but did not receive it): Thinking back to the time or times when you wanted to get professional help for stress, emotional, alcohol, drug, or family problems but did not, which of the following concerns kept you from getting professional help? Please select yes or no for each concern listed. [If this is not the respondent's first time completing the survey, insert the time qualifier "since (insert month and year of previous survey administration)" after "family problems…".]

Answer categories are:

1. Yes
2. No
99. Refused

1. Not knowing where to get help or who to see
2. Difficulty arranging transportation to treatment
3. Difficulty getting child care or time off of work
4. Difficulty scheduling an appointment
5. Difficulty paying for mental health treatment
6. Believing that the mental health treatments available to you are not very good
7. Medications having too many side-effects
8. Concerns about your treatment not being kept confidential
9. Concerns that your friends, family, or coworkers would respect you less
10. Concerns about losing contact or custody of your children
11. Concerns about harm being done to your career
12. Other reason not mentioned

Mental Health Treatment Preferences

MH5. If you wanted to get mental health care and could go to any type of provider free of charge, would you choose to go to: (programmer: allow for selection of only one choice)
1. a military health facility
2. a VA facility
3. a private, civilian provider
4. none of these
99. refused

MH6. If you wanted to get mental health care and could afford any of the following types of treatment, which one of the following treatments would you choose (programmer: allow for selection of only one option)?
   1. Medication prescribed by a health care provider
   2. Some type of counseling or talk therapy provided by a mental health specialist such as a psychiatrist, psychologist, counselor, or social worker
   3. Neither
   99. REF

FAMILY RELATIONSHIPS AND SOCIAL SUPPORT

Marriage/Significant Other

MF1. Are you…
   1. Married and living together
   2. Married and living separately by choice
   3. Married and living separately due to separate military assignments
   4. Living together as married
   5. Dating exclusively
   6. No current exclusive relationship [skip to MF3]
   99. REF SKIP TO MF3

[If this is not the respondent's first survey administration and the respondent's relationship status in the previous administration was one of the response options 1-5 for MF1 (i.e., involved in some sort of significant romantic relationship), clarify whether the person with whom they're involved is the same person or not: "Is the person with/to whom you are (insert relationship status, e.g., married and living together) now the same person with/to whom you were (insert relationship status at previous survey administration, e.g., married and living together) in (insert month and year of previous survey administration?" Response options are yes = 1, no = 2, DK = 98, REF = 99. If it is the same person, skip MF2 and go to MF3.]

MF2. How long have you been with this person? (Programmer: Show the following list of options:

1. less than one year (if respondent selects this option, take him/her to a new option to determine how many months [Question: "How many months have you been with this person?"]; show drop-down menu featuring options ranging from less than a month up to 11 months at 1-month increments)
2. 1 year
3. 2 years
4. 3 years
…continue to show 1-year increments up to 40 years

114

99. Refused

MF3.
a. How many children do you have by birth or adoption who depend on you for more than half of their financial support? (Response range: 0-20, 99 REF)
b. Please indicate the age of each child in years and whether he/she lives with you.
[Programmer: Please program age so that respondent selects it from a drop-down menu with the following response options:]
1. Less than 1 year old
2. 1 year old
3. 2 years old
4. 3 years old
…
24. 23 years old
25. older than 23
99. REF

	Age (years or months)	Lives with you (yes or no)
Child 1:		
Child 2:		
Child 3:		
…		

MF4. Who is living with you? From the list below, select each option that describes your relationship to each person who lives with you. [PROGRAMMER: Show checklist with a box next to each category of relationship so that respondent can select the box if that person lives with them or leave it unselected if not. If respondent has already said in MF1 that he/she is living with his/her spouse (MF1 = 1) or partner (MF1 = 4) or that he/she has dependents living with him/her in MF3, please program this question to include the word "else" in between "who" and "is", i.e., "Who else is living with you?" if we already know that someone lives with the respondent.]

1. My spouse or domestic partner [If MF1 = 1, 2, 3, 4, 5, or 6, skip this response option.]
2. My child(ren) [If respondent reported that at least one dependent lives with him/her in MF3, skip this response option.]
3. My parent(s)
4. My brother(s) and/or sister(s)
5. Other relatives
6. Others not related to me
7. Live by myself. [Programmer: If respondent has selected any of the boxes for response options 1-6, do not allow respondent to check this box. Program it so

that if the respondent selects this box, a prompt will appear that says something like, "You have already told us that you live with (fill blank with category of person selected); do you live with your (fill blank with category of person selected) OR do you live by yourself?]

MF5.1 Who most often helps you deal with problems that come up? From the following list, please select the option that best describes this person's relationship to you.
1. My spouse or domestic partner [If MF1 equals 5 (dating exclusively) or 6 (no current exclusive relationship), skip this option.]
2. Boyfriend or girlfriend
3. My child(ren)
4. My parent(s)
5. My brother(s) and/or sister(s)
6. Other relative
7. A friend
8. Not applicable
99. REF

[MF5.2 If this is not the respondent's first survey administration, and baseline MF5=follow up MF5, ask: Is this (insert name of primary supporter nominated in most recent survey administration), the same person that you mentioned the last time you completed this survey? (Response options: 1 = yes, 2 = no, 98 = DK, 99 = REF.)

MF6. Taking things altogether, how satisfied are you with (insert "your marriage" if the person is married OR "the relationship you have with the person who most often helps you deal with problems" if person is not married)? [Please program this question so that respondents who are not married (i.e., MF1 is not equal to 1, 2, or 3) and who select not applicable or refuse to answer MF5.1, i.e., no primary supporter, are skipped out of it. If this is not the respondent's first survey administration and the respondent indicated a different primary supporter in MF5 than the primary supporter they indicated in the previous survey administration, ask about "the relationship you have with the person who currently most often helps you deal with problems."]

[Response options include:]

Very satisfied......................1
Somewhat satisfied.................2
Neutral............................3
Somewhat dissatisfied.............4
Very dissatisfied..................5
Refuse............................ 99

116

Social Support

Now you are going to be asked some questions about support that you may or may not be able to get from different people in your life. For each of the following statements, select the choice that indicates how you feel.

Response options:
1. Strongly disagree
2. Disagree
3. Agree
4. Strongly agree
99. REF

1. There are people I can depend on to help me if I really need it.
2. I feel that I do not have close personal relationships with other people.
3. If something went wrong, no one would come to my assistance.
4. I have close relationships that provide me with a sense of emotional security and well-being.
5. I feel a strong emotional bond with at least one other person.
6. There is no one I can depend on for aid if I really need it.
7. There is no one with whom I have intimacy.
8. There are people I can count on in an emergency.

WORK AND CAREER

WC1. What is your current work status? Are you…
1. Working full-time, (go to WC2)
2. Working part-time, (go to WC2)

(If respondent endorses any of the options below, skip
Presenteeism/Absenteeism section.)
3. Unemployed and looking for work,
4. Unemployed and not looking for work,
5. Disabled and not working,
6. Full-time student,
7. Part-time student
8. Homemaker
9. Retired
98. DK
99. REF

Presenteeism/Absenteeism

[If working full (WC1 = 1) or part time (WC1 = 2)]

WC2. About how many hours altogether did you work in the past 7 days? (If
more than 97, enter 97.)

I Number of hours (00-97)

WC3. How many hours does your employer expect you to work in a typical 7-day
week? (If it varies, estimate the average. If more than 97, enter 97.)

I Number of hours (00-97)

WC4. Now please think of your work experiences over the past 4 weeks (28
days). You are going to be asked some questions about the number of days you
spent in different work situations.

In the past 4 weeks (28 days), how many days did you...[Programmer: Don't
allow the respondent to enter more than 28 days for WC4a-e—program a
message that asks for a number in between 0 and 28 if the respondent tries to
enter a number greater than 28.]

	Number of days (00-28)
WC4a. ...miss an **<u>entire</u>** work day because of problems with your physical or mental health? (Please include only days missed for your own health, not someone else's health.)	
WC4b. ...miss an **<u>entire</u>** work day for any other reason (including vacation)?	
WC4c. ...miss **part** of a work day because of problems with your physical or mental health? (Please include only days missed for your own health, not someone else's health.)	
WC4d. ...miss **part** of a work day for any other reason (including vacation)?	
WC4e. ...come in early, go home late, or work on your day off?	

WC5. On a scale from 0 to 10 where 0 is the worst job performance anyone could have at your job and 10 is the performance of a top worker, how would you rate the usual performance of <u>most</u> workers in a job similar to yours?

Worst Performance										*Top* Performance
0	1	2	3	4	5	6	7	8	9	10
☐	☐	☐	☐	☐	☐	☐	☐	☐	☐	☐

WC6. Using the same 0-to-10 scale, how would you rate your usual job performance over the past year or two?

Worst Performance										*Top* Performance
0	1	2	3	4	5	6	7	8	9	10
☐	☐	☐	☐	☐	☐	☐	☐	☐	☐	☐

WC7. Using the same 0-to-10 scale, how would you rate your overall job performance on the days you worked during the past 4 weeks (28 days)?

Worst Performance										*Top* Performance
0	1	2	3	4	5	6	7	8	9	10
☐	☐	☐	☐	☐	☐	☐	☐	☐	☐	☐

Employability

For some people work is just a way to get money, it's something they have to put up with. For others, work is the center of their life, something that really matters to them. The following items ask about your reactions to work in general, not simply your present paid job or paid jobs you have had in the past.

Please indicate how strongly you agree or disagree with each of the following statements.

Response options: [Programmer: For items WC8-WC13, please show a scale ranging from 1 to 5 with "disagree a lot" over the 1 and "agree a lot" over the 5.]

1. Disagree a lot
2.
3.
4.
5. Agree a lot
99. Refused

WC8. Even if I won a great deal of money in the lottery I would continue to work somewhere. On a scale of 1 through 5, where 1=disagree a lot and 5= agree a lot, how much do you agree or disagree?

WC9. Having a job is very important to me. On a scale of 1 through 5, where 1=disagree a lot and 5= agree a lot, how much do you agree or disagree?

WC10. I would hate to be getting employment handouts. On a scale of 1 through 5, where 1=disagree a lot and 5= agree a lot, how much do you agree or disagree?

WC11. I would soon get very bored if I had no work to do. On a scale of 1 through 5, where 1=disagree a lot and 5= agree a lot, how much do you agree or disagree?

WC12. The most important things that happen to me involve work. On a scale of 1 through 5, where 1=disagree a lot and 5= agree a lot, how much do you agree or disagree?

WC13. If the unemployment benefit was really high I would still prefer to work. On a scale of 1 through 5, where 1=disagree a lot and 5= agree a lot, how much do you agree or disagree?

Job Satisfaction

[If response to WC1 is employed full-time (WC1 = 1) or part-time (WC1 = 2), ask]:

WC14. How satisfied are you with your job in general?

Are you:
>   1 = very dissatisfied
>   2 = dissatisfied
>   3 = can't decide if I am satisfied or not
>   4 = satisfied
>   5 = very satisfied
>   99 = REF

Barriers to Employment

If respondent answered "Unemployed and looking for work" or "Disabled and not working" to question WC1, ask:

WC15. Which of the following make it difficult for you to obtain employment? Please select yes or no for each.

Response options include:
1. Yes
2. No
99. REF

Choose ALL that apply.

1. Not qualified-lack education
2. Not qualified-lack work history
3. Not enough pay
4. Do not know about available jobs
5. Family prefers I stay at home
6. Would lose financial benefits (e.g. disability benefits)
7. Would lose medical benefits
8. Pursuing an education
9. Do not have good transportation
10. Not physically capable
11. Cannot pass background checks due to criminal history
12. No one will hire me because of my injury or disability
13. I do not have the tools or knowledge to translate my military skills to the civilian workforce
14. I feel uncomfortable or get anxious when thinking about working in the civilian workplace

15. I lack confidence in myself and my abilities
16. Due to my long and/or multiple deployments, I feel behind compared to my peer civilian counterparts

Vocational Rehabilitation Services

Now I would like to ask you some questions about vocational rehabilitation services you might have received since returning from your most recent deployment. Vocational rehabilitation services are designed to help you return to work after an injury. These services include occupational therapy, physical therapy, personal adjustment training, training in self-care, training in vocational, college, or job seeking skills, employment assistance.

WC16. Have you received any vocational rehabilitation services from ... [If this is not the respondent's first survey administration, begin the sentence with "since (insert month and year of most recent survey administration)" have you received....]

	Yes	No	Does Not Apply	RF
a. A military program?	1	2	3	99
b. A Veterans Affairs (VA) program?	1	2	3	99
c. Another program?	1	2	3	99

ECONOMIC SITUATION

Income and Disability Compensation

ID1. What is your household's total annual income from all sources before taxes in 2010? Include money from jobs, social security, retirement income, disability payments, unemployment payments, public assistance, investments and so forth. [For survey administrations that take place one year or more after January 1, 2011, update year as needed to reflect the most recent year for which annual income is known.]

    1. Less than $10,000
    2. 10,000 to less than $20,000
    3. 20,000 to less than $30,000
    4. 30,000 to less than $40,000__
    5. 40,000 to less than $50,000
    6. 50,000 to less than $75,000
    7. 75,000 to less than $100,000
    8. $100,000 or more
  98. dk
  99. refused_____

ID2. Including yourself, how many people in your household are supported by your total
    household income? _____(1-15+, 99 REF)

Financial Strain

The next few questions are about your finances. Please answer the following question on a scale of 1 (not at all difficult) to 5 (extremely difficult or impossible) (DK = 98, REF = 99).

FS1. How difficult is it for you to live on your total household income right now? [Response options:]
1 = not at all difficult
2
3
4
5 = extremely difficult or impossible
99. REF

FS2. In the next two months, how much do you think that you or other members of your household will experience problems such as not having a home, or not enough food or medical care? Please answer this question on a scale of 1 (not at all) to 5 (a great deal).

[Response options:]
1 = not at all
2
3
4
5 = a great deal
99. REF

FS3. In the next two months, how much do you think you will have to reduce your lifestyle to the bare necessities? Please answer this question on a scale of 1 (not at all) to 5 (a great deal).

[Response options:]
1 = not at all
2
3
4
5 = a great deal
99. REF

FS4. Who has primary responsibility for managing your finances—for example, making sure bills are paid on time, deciding how to spend money, etc.?
1. Self
2. Spouse or partner
3. Parent
4. Child(ren)
5. Other relative, such as sibling, aunt, uncle
6. Other
99. REF

Housing

H1. Have you **ever** spent the night in any of the following places during your lifetime **because you had no regular place to stay**, like your own house, apartment, or room (including military housing), or in the home of a family member or friend? [If this is not the respondent's first survey administration, delete the word "ever" and begin the sentence with "Since (insert month and year of most recent survey administration) …"]

Response options:
1. Yes
2. No (skip to next section)
99. REF (skip to next section)

a) a transitional shelter or program
b) a mission or homeless shelter
c) a church or chapel (but not in a bed)
d) an all-night theater or other indoor public place
e) an abandoned building
f) a car or other vehicle
g) the street or in some other outdoor place

[If respondent answers no (2) to all of the above (a-g), skip the rest of the Housing section. If respondent answers yes (1) to any of the above (a-g) and this is the respondent's first survey administration, ask H2 and H3; otherwise, skip to H4.]

H2. When was the **first time** you ever spent the night in any of those places because you had no regular place to stay? That is, when did your stay the first time begin? Please provide the month and year of the first time you stayed in any of those places.
[Programmer: List drop-down menu for month that includes all months of the year and a drop-down menu for year that includes all years going all the way back to 1940.]

H3. When was the **last** time you had to spend the night in any one of those places? That is, when did that last time end? Please provide the month and year of the last time you stayed in any of those places. [If respondent gives a response to this question that is inconsistent with the response to H2, i.e., he/she says the last time took place before the first time, have prompt appear to query respondent for an internally consistent response: "Are you sure that the last time you lived in one of those places was April 2010? You said in response to an earlier question that the first time you lived in one of those places was June 2010. Do you want to change the answers you've given?" Program a response option for the respondent to indicate yes (to change answers) or no (to proceed with the rest of the survey). When the respondent selects "yes," he/she should be taken back to the original screen and allowed to re-enter responses. If responses to H2 and H3 indicate that the last time the respondent spent the night in any of those places occurred less than 6 months ago, ask H4; otherwise, skip to H5.]

[Programmer: List drop-down menu for month that includes all months of the year and a drop-down menu for year that includes all years going all the way back to 1940. Also include a response option for "still living in one of those places"—e.g., OR Are you still living in one of those places?]

H4. How much time altogether have you spent in any of these places during the last 6 months, since [FILL DATE]? [If this is not the respondent's first survey administration, replace the number "6" with the number of months in between this survey administration and the previous administration and fill the date with the month and year of the previous administration.]
Response options:
1. Less than 1 week
2. 1 week
3. 2 weeks
4. 3 weeks
5. 1 month
6. 2 months
7. 3 months
8. 4 months
9. 5 months
10. 6 months
99. REF

Current living situation

H5. How long have you lived at your current place of residence?

Response options:
1. Less than 1 year
2. 1 year
3. 2 years
4. 3 years
5...4-50 years listed at 1-year increments
99. REF

H6. The following list contains places where you might have lived during the past six months, that is, since [FILL DATE]. For each place, please select "yes" if you have lived there since [FILL DATE] and "no"' if you have not. Include any of the places you reported earlier and where you're living now. [Please program a skip pattern such that respondents who said "no" in H1 to ever having lived in the corresponding place for options o-u of H6 are not asked if they've lived in one of these places in the past 6 months. For example, if a respondent says in H1 that he/she has never spent the night in a transitional shelter or program, he/she would be skipped out of option "o" (transitional shelter or program) in H6 (but would still be read all of the other housing options to which he/she has not already said no). Please do not display the section headings, e.g., "HOUSING." If this is not the respondent's first survey administration, replace the number "6" with the number of months in between this survey administration and the previous administration.]

1. Yes
2. No
99. REF

HOUSING
a) Apartment or home of your own (including rented)
b) A partner's home, apartment or room
c) Family's home, apartment or room
d) Friend's home, apartment or room

HOTEL/MOTEL
e) In hotel or motel that you paid for
f) In hotel or motel partner paid for
g) In hotel or motel family or friends paid for
h) In hotel or motel paid for with voucher

SPECIALIZED HOUSING
(Ask i only if respondent is woman.)
i) A special facility or shelter for battered women
j) A boarding house, halfway house, board and care facility group home, or sober living shelter

TREATMENT OR CORRECTIONAL FACILITY OR HOSPITAL
k) Residential alcohol or drug treatment program or detox
l) Psychiatric hospital or drug treatment inpatient facility
m) Hospital (for medical/physical health reasons)
n) Jail or prison
o) Transitional shelter or program

HOMELESS SETTING
p) Mission or homeless shelter

q) Church or chapel (but not in a bed)
r) All night theater, other indoor public place
s) Abandoned building
t) Car, or other vehicle
u) Street, or other outdoor vehicle (including homeless encampment)

H6a. Where are you currently living? (Programmer: After respondent goes through list and has selected yes or no for each, display list of places that the respondent says they have lived in the past six months and ask, "Which of the following places is your current residence?")

[PROGRAMMER: If respondent selects one of the places under the "HOTEL/MOTEL" or "HOMELESS SETTING" categories in response to H6, ask H7; if respondent selected multiple options under either of these categories, ask H7 for each option selected. If the respondent did not select any options in the "HOMELESS SETTING" or "HOTEL/MOTEL" categories in H6, skip to H8]

H7. Did you stay in a [Fill option selected] because you had no regular place to stay, like your own house, apartment, or room or in the home of a family member or friend?" (Only count as homeless if respondent answers yes to this item.)

1. Yes
2. No
99. REF

H8. Do you consider yourself to have been homeless at any time during the past six months? [If this is not the respondent's first survey administration, replace the number "6" with the number of months in between this survey administration and the previous administration.]

1. Yes
2. No
99. REF

(Ask H9 only if respondent endorses any of the above places other than k, l, m, or n that are indicative of being at-risk for homelessness or homeless)

H9. Please read the following list of possible reasons why people might not live in an apartment or home that they (and/or their partner) own or rent. Then select the main reason that you do not currently live in an apartment or home that you (and/or your partner) own or rent. (Programmer: include phrase "and/or your partner" only if respondent indicated that they have a partner, i.e., selected response option 1, 2, 3, 4, or 5 to MF1; allow respondent to select only one choice).

1. Saving money for my own place
2. Hiding from creditors
3. Cannot afford it
4. House foreclosed on
5. Enjoy staying with friends/family (programmer: allow for selection of this option only if respondent indicated in response to a previous question that his/her current place of residence is a family member or friend's home, apartment, or room)
6. Left housing due to relationship difficulties with living companions
7. Hard to find quality housing
99. REF

PHYSICAL HEALTH

Physical Functioning (SF-36)

Physical Health

PH1. In general, would you say your health is:

Excellent............. 1
Very good........... 2
Good................... 3
Fair 4
Poor.................... 5
REF.................99

PH2. During the past 4 weeks, have you had any of the following problems with your work or other regular daily activities as a result of your physical health?

[INSERT GRID – COLUMNS:]
1. Yes
2. No
99. Refused

1. Cut down the amount of time you spent on work or other activities
2. Accomplished less than you would like
3. Were limited in the kind of work or other activities
4. Had difficulty performing the work or other activities (for example, it took extra effort)

C. Additional Results

Below in tabular form are additional descriptive results from our baseline survey that supplement the findings from the rest of the document. We begin by presenting the detailed comparison of our respondents to the population (Table C.1). We follow with additional health-related information, further details on family demographics and social situation. We end with additional detail on work and financial situation.

Table C.1. Comparison of Medically Retired and Active-duty Airmen Served by the Air Force Wounded Warrior Program to Survey Completers (N = 872)

Characteristic	Population (N = 872)		Survey Completers (N = 459)			
	N	Percentage	N	Percentage	95% CI LL	95% CI UL
Component						
Active	618	70.9	320	69.7	65.5	73.9
Air Force Reserve	120	13.8	65	14.2	11.0	17.4
Traditional Reservist	88	73.3	45	69.2	58.0	80.5
Air National Guard	132	15.1	73	15.9	12.6	19.3
Drill (versus other)	109	82.6	61	83.6	75.1	92.1
AFSC						
1	162	18.6	89	19.4	15.8	23.0
2	218	25.0	117	25.5	21.5	29.5
3	352	40.4	171	37.3	32.8	41.7
4	93	10.7	58	12.6	9.6	15.7
Other (5–9)	45	5.2	23	5.0	3.0	7.0
Enlisted	773	88.7	393	85.6	82.4	88.8
Number of deployments						
0	88	10.1	47	10.2	7.5	13.0
1	335	38.4	169	36.8	32.4	41.2
2	232	26.6	119	25.9	21.9	29.9
3	121	13.9	69	15.0	11.8	18.3
4 or more	96	11.0	55	12.0	9.0	15.0

Table C.1—Continued

Characteristic	Population (N = 872)		Survey Completers (N = 459)			
	N	Percentage	N	Percentage	95% CI LL	95% CI UL
Operation supported by most recent deployment						
Operation Enduring Freedom	274	31.4	142	30.9	26.7	35.2
Operation Iraqi Freedom	492	56.4	259	56.4	51.9	61.0
Other	102	11.7	57	12.4	9.4	15.4
Retired	567	65.0	284	61.9	57.4	66.3
Male	744	85.3	394	85.8	82.7	89.0
Race/ethnicity						
White	669	76.7	357	77.78	74.0	81.6
Hispanic	83	9.5	48	10.46	7.7	13.3
Black	70	8.0	31	6.75	4.5	9.1
Other	29	3.3	11	2.40	1.0	3.8
College degree or higher	144	16.5	96	20.92	17.2	24.6
	M	SD	M	SD	95% CI LL	95% CI UL
Length of most recent deployment (months)	4.48	2.78	4.63	2.82	4.37	4.89
Years since return from most recent deployment	4.18	2.07	4.19	2.07	3.99	4.39
Total active years in the military (active duty only)	11.03	6.32	12.38	6.63	11.65	13.11
Years since most recent Air Force separation	1.84	2.19	1.79	2.23	1.58	1.99
Age	34.87	8.77	36.38	9.08	35.54	37.21

NOTES: CI = confidence interval; LL = lower limit; UL = upper limit. For "Traditional Reservist," the denominator for the percentage listed is the number of Air Force Reservists. For "Drill (versus other)," the denominator for the percentage listed is the number of airmen in the Air National Guard. The "other" category for "operation supported by most recent deployment" includes airmen who never deployed.

As illustrated above, differences between our respondents and the overall population of AFW2 enrollees (excluding separatees) were minimal. In the few cases where they were statistically significant (college degree or higher, total active years in the military, and age) they were not substantively meaningful. We next offer further detailed survey responses to health care–related items.

Health Care

Respondents' health insurance coverage other than through VA or TRICARE was assessed (all respondents in the sample are eligible for VA and/or TRICARE). As shown in Table C.2, just over one-quarter of respondents reported that they were currently covered by health insurance other than VA or TRICARE. Similarly, just over a quarter of respondents had obtained reduced costs of health insurance for themselves or their family members since returning from their most recent deployment or deployment-related activities.

Table C.2. Health Insurance Status (N = 459)

	N	Percentage	95% CI LL	95% CI UL
Currently covered by health insurance other than VA or TRICARE	120	26.1	22.1	30.2
Reduced costs of health insurance for airman or his/her family members received since return from most recent deployment or deployment-related activities	116	25.3	21.3	29.3

NOTES: CI = confidence interval; LL = lower limit; UL = upper limit.

More than three-quarters of respondents reported having received prescription medication or talk therapy during the past year, indicating that these types of treatment were utilized by nearly equal proportions of respondents. Just over a third of respondents reported having received a form of mental health treatment other than prescription medication or talk therapy. (See Table C.3.)

Slightly more than two-thirds of respondents reported having received both prescription medication and talk therapy during the past year. Less than 10 percent of the sample reported having received only medication or only talk therapy during the past year. Thus, receipt of medication and talk therapy at some point during the past year was fairly typical for this sample.

Table C.3. Specific Details on Mental Health Services (N = 459)

	N	Percentage	95% CI LL	95% CI UL
Mental health services were desired but not obtained	199	43.4	38.8	47.9
Any mental health services received	397	86.5	83.4	89.6
Medication prescribed for mental health problems	360	78.4	74.7	82.2
Received therapy for mental health problems	358	78.0	74.2	81.8
Some other treatment received	174	37.9	33.5	42.4
Co-occurrence of receiving medication and therapy for mental health problems				
Neither medication nor therapy received	65	14.2	11.0	17.4
Only medication received	36	7.8	5.4	10.3
Only therapy received	34	7.4	5.0	9.8
Both medication and therapy received	324	70.6	66.4	74.8
Mental health services setting				
Military treatment facility	221	48.2	43.6	52.7
VHA facility	266	58.0	53.4	62.5
Civilian facility	231	50.3	45.8	54.9

Family and Social Characteristics

We also offer further detail on family and social characteristics. Approximately a third of respondents did not have any dependents under the age of 23 (see Table C.4). Nearly half of respondents had one or two dependents, and slightly less than one-fifth had three or more dependents. Of respondents who had one or more dependents, roughly one-quarter had dependents between the ages of five and nine or between the ages of 10 and 14. Just over one-fifth of respondents had dependents who were four years old or younger, and just under one-fifth of respondents had dependents in middle to late adolescence (i.e., 15 to 19 years old). Slightly more than 10 percent of respondents had dependents older than 19.

Table C.4. Number and Ages of Dependents

Number of Dependents (N = 459)	N	Percentage	95% CI LL	95% CI UL
0	156	34.0	29.7	38.3
1	93	20.3	16.6	23.9
2	125	27.2	23.2	31.3
3 or more	80	17.4	14.0	20.9
Age of Dependents (N = 298)				
0-4 years old	97	21.1	17.4	24.9
5-9 years old	122	26.6	22.5	30.6
10-14 years old	117	25.5	21.5	29.5
15-19 years old	83	18.1	14.6	21.6
20 years old or older	55	12.0	9.0	15.0

NOTES: CI = confidence interval; LL = lower limit; UL = upper limit. Percentages for ages of dependents do not sum to 100 because of respondents who have more than one child and are therefore counted in more than one category.

134

Nearly two-thirds of respondents indicated that they reside with their spouse or domestic partner, and just over half reported residing with their children. A minority of respondents (less than 20 percent) reported living alone. Minorities of respondents (i.e., roughly 10 percent or less) reported living with their parents, siblings, other relatives, or others not related to them. Detailed results on household structure are provided in Table C.5.

Table C.5. Household Structure (N = 459)

Household Member(s)	N	Percentage	95% CI LL	95% CI UL
Spouse or domestic partner	302	65.8	61.5	70.1
Children	260	56.6	52.1	61.2
Lives alone	71	15.5	12.2	18.8
Parent(s)/Parent(s)-in-law	42	9.2	6.5	11.8
Brother(s)/brother(s)-in-law and/or sister(s)/sister(s)-in-law	19	4.1	2.3	6.0
Other relatives	16	3.5	1.8	5.2
Others not related to respondent	50	10.9	8.0	13.7

NOTES: CI = confidence interval; LL = lower limit; UL = upper limit.

Respondents also reported the levels of social support that they perceive to be available to them from different people in their lives. Two dimensions of social support were assessed with subscales of the Social Provisions Scale (SPS; Cutrona and Russell, 1987): (1) Reliable Alliance, which refers to the availability of instrumental support (e.g., people to depend on in an emergency), and (2) Attachment, which refers to the availability of emotional support from and intimacy with other people. On average, respondents scored closer to the high end of both the Reliable Alliance and Attachment subscales than the low end, suggesting that respondents tended to perceive that both instrumental and emotional support were generally available to them. (See Table C.6.)

Table C.6. Perceived Social Support Available to Airman from Different People in His/Her Life (N = 459)

Social Support Dimension	M	SD	95% CI LL	95% CI UL
Reliable alliance	12.47	2.68	12.22	12.71
Attachment	11.02	2.98	10.74	11.30

NOTES: M = mean; SD = standard deviation; CI = confidence interval; LL = lower limit; UL = upper limit. Possible scores on the Reliable Alliance and Attachment subscales range from 4 to 16. Higher scores on the Reliable Alliance subscale indicate that the airman perceives greater availability of instrumental support (e.g., help in an emergency) from people in his or her life. Higher scores on the Attachment subscale indicate that the airman perceives greater availability of emotional support from and intimacy with people in his or her life.

Work and Finances

Work involvement is based on a measure developed by Warr et al. (1979) to gauge how central work is perceived to be and may be used as a predictor of job seeking behaviors among the unemployed. These questions were asked of all airmen, regardless of employment status. There are six items; a score of 6 means that respondents "disagree a lot" with all of the statements describing various ways work may be viewed as important, while a score of 30 means that respondents consistently "agree a lot" with statements indicating that work is very central to their lives. On average, airmen agree that work is more important and central than not in their lives, as shown in Table C.7. The difference in the average rating of work involvement between those classified as employed at least part time and whose who were not employed was not significant, $t(447) = 0.671$, $p = 0.50$, indicating that among these airmen work involvement was not related to their employment status.

Table C.7. Work Involvement (N = 459)

	M	SD	95% CI LL	95% CI UL
Work involvement	21.27	6.48	20.67	21.87

NOTES: M = mean; SD = standard deviation; CI = confidence interval; LL = lower limit; UL = upper limit. Possible and observed scores on the Work Involvement scale ranged from 6 to 30, with higher scores indicating more positive attitudes toward work.

Although only 8.5 percent of airmen indicated that they were currently pursuing studies, 34 percent, or just over one-third of respondents, indicated that they had received some form of financial aid for education since their deployment or deployment-related activities (see Table C.8). When asked whether they perceived financial aid to be helpful, regardless of whether they had themselves taken advantage of these benefits, the response was quite positive with approximately 84 percent indicating that they perceived it as helpful. With regard to job training, the response was only somewhat less positive, with about 74 percent indicating they felt these types of benefits to be helpful.

Table C.8. Financial Aid for Education and Job Training (N = 459)

	N	Percentage	95% CI LL	95% CI UL
Financial aid for education received since deployment or deployment-related activities	156	34.0	29.7	38.3
Perceived helpfulness of financial aid for education (regardless of whether financial aid for education has been received)	385	83.9	80.5	87.2
Perceived helpfulness of job training (regardless of whether job training has been received)	338	73.6	69.6	77.7

NOTES: CI = confidence interval; LL = lower limit; UL = upper limit.

Airmen were asked if they had received vocational rehabilitation services since their return. Specifically, they were asked if they had received such services via a military program, via a VA program, or via some other program. Approximately 32 percent, or one-third, had received some form of such services, with the largest number indicating this was through the VA (19.61 percent). Of those who had received some vocational rehabilitation services, the majority (71.72 percent) had received them from only one source, while the remainder indicated services from multiple sources. (See Table C.9.)

Table C.9. Vocational Rehabilitation Services Utilization (N = 459)

	N	Percentage	95% CI LL	95% CI UL
Vocational rehabilitation services received	145	31.6	27.3	35.8
Setting in which services were received				
Military program	74	16.1	12.8	19.5
Veterans Affairs program	90	19.6	16.0	23.2
Another program	24	5.2	3.2	7.3

NOTES: CI = confidence interval; LL = lower limit; UL = upper limit.

References

Achtmeyer, Carol, and Katharine Bradley, "Using AUDIT-C Alcohol Screening Data in VA Research: Interpretation, Strengths, Limitations, and Sources," Northwest HSR&D Center of Excellence, VA Puget Sound, Substance Use Disorders QUERI, Center of Excellence in Substance Abuse Treatment and Education, Department of Medicine, University of Washington, March 2011. As of January 14, 2014: http://www.hsrd.research.va.gov/for_researchers/cyber_seminars/archives/vci-031511.pdf

Adler, A. B., B. T. Litz, C. A. Castro, M. Suvak, J. L. Thomas, L. Burrell, D. McGurk, K.M. Wright, and P.D. Bliese, "A group randomized trial of critical incident stress debriefing provided to US peacekeepers," *Journal of Traumatic Stress*, Vol. 21, 2008, pp. 253–263.

Air Force Instruction 41-210, *Tricare Operations and Patient Administration Functions,* Washington, D.C.: Department of the Air Force, June 6, 2012. As of January 10, 2014: http://static.e-publishing.af.mil/production/1/af_sg/publication/afi41-210/afi41-210.pdf

Air Force Instruction 48-123, *Medical Examinations and Standards,* September 24, 2009, Incorporating Through Change 2, October 18, 2011, Air Force Materiel Command Supplement, July 19, 2012, Washington, D.C.: Department of the Air Force. As of January 10, 2014: http://static.e-publishing.af.mil/production/1/afmc/publication/afi48-123_afmcsup_i/afi48-123_afmcsup_i.pdf

Air Force Wounded Warriors, "AFW2 Eligibility," undated. As of January 10, 2014: http://www.woundedwarrior.af.mil/questions/topic.asp?id=1372

American Psychiatric Association, *Diagnostic and Statistical Manual of Mental Disorders,* 4th ed., Washington, D.C.: American Psychiatric Associates, 1994.

American Psychiatric Association, *Publication Manual of the American Psychological Association,* 5th ed., Washington, D.C.: American Psychiatric Associates, 2001.

Anderson, I. M., "Selective Serotonin Reuptake Inhibitors Versus Tricyclic Antidepressants: A Meta-Analysis of Efficacy and Tolerability," *Journal of Affective Disorders*, Vol. 58, 2000, pp. 19–36.

Arciniegas, D. B., C. A. Anderson, J. Topkoff, and T. W. McAllister, "Mild Traumatic Brain Injury: A Neuropsychiatric Approach to Diagnosis, Evaluation, and Treatment," *Neuropsychiatric Disease and Treatment*, Vol. 1, No. 4, 2005, pp. 311–327.

Arvey, Richard D., Itzhak Harpaz, and Hui Liao, "Work Centrality and Post-Award Work Behavior of Lottery Winners," *The Journal of Psychology: Interdisciplinary and Applied*, Vol. 138, No. 5, 2010, pp. 404–420.

Ball, K., J. D. Edwards, and L. A. Ross, "The Impact of Speed of Processing Training on Cognitive and Everyday Functions," *Journals of Gerontology: SERIES B-Psychological Sciences and Social Sciences*, Vol. 62, No. I, 2007, pp. 19–31.

Banerjee, Souvik, Pinka Chatterji, and Kajal Lahiri, "Effects of Psychiatric Disorders on Labor Market Outcomes: A Latent Variable Approach Using Multiple Clinical Indicators," CESifo Working Paper Series No. 4260, May 2013.

Baruch, Y., "Response Rate in Academic Studies—A Comparative Analysis," *Human Relations,* Vol. 52, 1999, pp. 421–438.

Berglass, Nancy, and Margaret Harrell, *Well After Service: Veteran Reintegration and American Communities*, Washington, D.C.: Center for a New American Security, 2012.

Besterman-Dahan, K., S. Barnett, E. Hickling, C. Elnitsky, J. Lind, J. Skvoretz, and N. Antinori, "Bearing the Burden: Deployment Stress Among Army National Guard Chaplains," *Journal of Health Care Chaplain*, Vol. 18, No. 3–4, 2012, pp. 133–150.

Besterman-Dahan, K., S. W. Gibbons, S. D. Barnett, and E. J. Hickling, "The Role of Military Chaplains in Mental Health Care of the Deployed Service Member," *Military Medicine*, Vol. 177, No. 9, 2012, pp. 1028–1033.

Blanchard, E. B., E. J. Hickling, A. J. Vollmer, W. R. Loos, T. C. Buckley, and J. Jaccard, "Short-Term Follow-Up of Post-Traumatic Stress Symptoms in Motor Vehicle Accident Victims," *Behavior Research and Therapy*, Vol. 33, No. 4, 1995, pp. 369–377.

Blanchard, E. B., J. Jones-Alexander, T. C. Buckley, and C. A. Forneris, "Psychometric Properties of the PTSD Checklist (PCL)," *Behavior Research and Therapy*, Vol. 34, No. 8, 1996, pp. 669–673.

Bliese, Paul D., Kathleen M. Wright, Amy B. Adler, Jeffrey L. Thomas, and Charles W. Hoge, "Timing of Postcombat Mental Health Assessments," *Psychological Services*, Vol. 4, No. 3, 2007, pp. 141–148.

Bohnert, A. S., C. P. Bradshaw, and C. A. Latkin, "A Social Network Perspective on Heroin and Cocaine Use Among Adults: Evidence of Bidirectional Influences," *Addiction*, Vol. 107, 2009, pp. 1210–1218.

Bonanno, G. A., "Loss, Trauma, and Human Resilience: Have We Underestimated the Human Capacity to Thrive After Extremely Aversive Events?" *American Psychologist*, Vol. 59, 2004, pp. 20–28.

Bonanno, G. A., "Resilience in the Face of Potential Trauma," *Current Directions in Psychological Science*, Vol. 14, 2005, pp. 135–138.

Bond, Gary R., Sandra G. Resnick, Robert E. Drak, Haiyi Xie, Gregory J. McHugo, and Richard R. Bebout, "Does Competitive Employment Improve Nonvocational Outcomes for People With Severe Mental Illness?" *Journal of Consulting and Clinical Psychology*, Vol. 69, No. 3, 2001, pp. 489–501.

Bond, G. R., "Supported Employment: Evidence for an Evidence-Based Practice," *Psychiatric Rehabilitation Journal*, Vol. 27, 2004, pp. 345–358.

Bradley, Rebekah, Jamelle Greene, Eric Russ, Lissa Dutra, and Drew Westen, "A Multidimensional Meta-Analysis of Psychotherapy for PTSD," *American Journal of Psychiatry*, Vol. 162, No. 2, 2005, pp. 214–227.

Bray, R. M., M. R. Pemberton, M. E. Lane, L. L. Hourani, M. J. Mattiko, and L. A. Babeu, "Substance Use and Mental Health Trends Among U.S. Military Active Duty Personnel: Key Findings from the 2008 DoD Health Behavior Survey," *Military Medicine*, Vol. 175, No. 6, 2010, pp. 390–399.

Brazier, J. E., R. Harper, N. M. Jones, A. O'Cathain, K. J. Thomas, T. Usherwood, and L. Westlake, "Validating the SF-36 Health Survey Questionnaire: New Outcome Measure for Primary Care," *British Medical Journal*, Vol. 305, July 18, 1992, pp. 160–164.

Brewin, Chris B., Bernice Andrews, and John D. Valentine, "Meta-Analysis of Risk Factors for Posttraumatic Stress Disorder in Trauma-Exposed Adults," *Journal of Consulting and Clinical Psychology*, Vol. 68, No. 5, 2000, pp. 748–766.

Brewin, C. R., "Systematic Review of Screening Instruments for Adults at Risk of PTSD," *Journal of Traumatic Stress*, Vol. 18, No. 1, 2005, pp. 53–62.

Brown, Harriet, "Looking for Evidence That Therapy Works," *NYTimes.com*, March 25, 2013. As of January 15, 2014:
http://well.blogs.nytimes.com/2013/03/25/looking-for-evidence-that-therapy-works/?_r=0

Buchwald, Dedra, Tsilke Pearlman, Jovine Umali, Karen Schmaling, and Wayne Katon, "Functional Status in Patients with Chronic Fatigue Syndrome, Other Fatiguing Illnesses, and Healthy Individuals," *American Journal of Medicine*, Vol. 101, No. 4, October 1996, pp. 364–370.

Bureau of Labor Statistics, "Databases, Tables, and Calculators by Subject," online, undated. As of April 11, 2013:
http://www.bls.gov/data

Bureau of Labor Statistics, "The Employment Situation—May 2013," June 2013. As of June 19, 2013:
http://www.bls.gov/news.release/pdf/empsit.pdf

Burnett-Ziegler, I., M. Ilgen, M. Valenstein, K. Zivin, L. Gorman, A. Blow, S. Duffy, and S. Chermack, "Prevalence and Correlates of Alcohol Misuse Among Returning Afghanistan and Iraq Veterans," *Addictive Behaviors*, Vol. 36, 2011, pp. 801–806.

Burnam, M. Audrey, Lisa S. Meredith, Todd C. Helmus, Rachel M. Burns, Robert A. Cox, Elizabeth D'Amico, Laurie T. Martin, Mary E. Vaiana, Kayla M. Williams, and Michael R. Yochelson, "Systems of Care: Challenges and Opportunities to Improve Access to High-Quality Care," in Terri Tanielian and Lisa H. Jaycox, eds., *Invisible Wounds of War: Psychological and Cognitive Injuries, Their Consequences, and Services to Assist Recovery,* Santa Monica, Calif.: RAND Corporation, MG-720-CCF, 2008, pp. 245–428. As of January 14, 2014:
http://www.rand.org/pubs/monographs/MG720

Burt, Martha, Laudan Y. Aron, and Edgar Lee, with Jesse Valente, *Helping America's Homeless: Emergency Shelter or Affordable Housing?* Washington, D.C.: The Urban Institute Press, 2001.

Bush, K., D. R. Kivlahan, M. B. McDonell, S. D. Fihn, and K. A. Bradley, "The AUDIT Alcohol Consumption Questions (AUDIT-C): An Effective Brief Screening Test for Problem Drinking. Ambulatory Care Quality Improvement Project (ACQUIP). Alcohol Use Disorders Identification Test," *Archives of Internal Medicine*, Vol. 148, No. 16, 1998, pp. 1789–1795.

Butler, Andrew C., Jason E. Chapman, Evan M. Forman, and Aaron T. Beck. "The Empirical Status of Cognitive-Behavioral Therapy: A Review of Meta-Analyses," *Clinical Psychology Review*, Vol. 26, 2006, pp. 17–31. As of January 14, 2014:
http://www.researchgate.net/publication/7566273_The_empirical_status_of_cognitive-behavioral_therapy_a_review_of_meta-analyses/links/0912f5040d085a6d5d000000

Campbell, D. G., B. L. Felker, C. F. Liu, E. M. Yano, J. E. Kirchner, D. Chan, L.V. Rubenstein, E.F. Chaney, "Prevalence of Depression-PTSD Comorbidity: Implications for Clinical Practice Guidelines and Primary Care-Based Interventions," *Journal of General Internal Medicine*, Vol. 22, No. 6, 2007, pp. 711–718.

Carroll, J. S., C. A. Meyer, J. Song, W. Li, T. R. Geistlinger, J. Eeckhoute, A. S. Brodsky, E. K. Keeton, K. C. Fertuck, G. F. Hall, Qianben Wang, Stefan Bekiranov, Victor Sementchenko, Edward A. Fox, Pamela A. Silver, Thosas R. Gingeras, Shirley Liu, and Myles Brown, "Genomewide Analysis of Estrogen Receptor Binding Sites," *Nature Genetics*, Vol. 38, 2006, pp. 1289–1297.

Cascalenda, N., J. C. Perry, and K. Looper, "Remission in Major Depressive Disorder: A Comparison of Pharmacotherapy, Psychotherapy, and Control Conditions," *American Journal of Psychiatry*, Vol. 159, 2002, pp. 1354–1360.

Chewning, B., and B. Sleath, "Medication Decision-Making and Management: A Client-Centered Model," *Social Science and Medicine*, Vol. 42, 1996, pp. 1299–1304.

Christensen, Brandon N., and Joanne Yaffe, "Factors Affecting Mental Health Service Utilization Among Deployed Military Personnel," *Military Medicine*, Vol. 177, No. 3, 2012, pp. 278–283.

Christensen, Eric, J. McMahon, E. Schaefer, T. Jaditz, and D. Harris, *Final Report for the Veterans' Disability Benefits Commission: Compensation, Survey Results, and Selected Topics*, Washington, D.C.: Center for Naval Analysis, 2007.

Cohen, Sheldon, "Social Relationships and Health," *American Psychologist*, Vol. 59, 2004, pp. 676–684.

Cohen, Sheldon, Benjamin H. Gottlieb, and Lynn G. Underwood, "Social Relationships and Health," in S. Cohen, L. Underwood, and B. Gottlieb, eds., *Measuring and Intervening in Social Support*, New York: Oxford University Press, 2000, pp. 3–25.

Cohen, Sheldon, and Thomas Ashby Wills, "Stress, Social Support, and the Buffering Hypothesis," *Psychological Bulletin*, Vol. 98, No. 2, 1985, pp. 310–357.

Colella, Adrienne J., and Susanne M. Bruyere, "Disability and Employment: New Directions for Industrial and Organizational Psychology," in *APA Handbook of Industrial and Organizational Psychology,* Washington, D.C.: American Psychological Association, 2010, pp. 473–503.

Cook, Judith, "Employment Barriers for Persons with Psychiatric Disabilities: Update of a Report for the President's Commission," *Psychiatric Services*, Vol. 57, No. 10, 2006, pp. 1391–1405.

Cooke, Betty D., Marilyn Martin Rossmann, Hamilton I. McCubbin, and Joan M. Patterson, "Examining the Definition and Assessment of Social Support: A Resource for Individuals and Families," *Family Relations*, Vol. 32, No. 2, 1988, pp. 211–216.

Corbiere, Marc, and Tania LeComte, "Vocational Services Offered to People with Severe Mental Services," *Journal of Mental Health*, Vol. 18, No. 1, 2009, pp. 38–50.

Corrigan, John D., and Thomas B. Cole, "Substance Use Disorders and Clinical Management of Traumatic Brain Injury and Posttraumatic Stress Disorder," *JAMA*, Vol. 300, No. 6, 2008, pp. 720–721.

Corrigan, P. W., K. T. Mueser, G. R. Bond, R. E. Drake, and P. Solomon, *Principles and Practice of Psychiatric Rehabilitation: An Empirical Approach,* New York: Guilford Press, 2007.

Cutrona, C. E., and D. W. Russell, "The Provisions of Social Relationships and Adaptation to Stress," *Advances in Personal Relationships*, Vol. 1, 1987, pp. 37–67.

Deegan, P. E., and R. E. Drake, "Shared Decision Making and Medication Management in the Recovery Process," *Psychiatric Services*, Vol. 57, 2006, pp. 1636–1639.

Defense Health Board Task Force on Mental Health, "An Achievable Vision: Report of the Department of Defense Task Force on Mental Health," June 2007. As of June 19, 2013:
http://www.health.mil/dhb/mhtf/mhtf-report-final.pdf

Defense Manpower Data Center, *2010 Military Family Life Project*, Arlington, Va.: Department of Defense, 2011.

Defense and Veterans Brain Injury Center, "DoD Numbers for Traumatic Brain Injury," online, data as of May 9, 2013. As of January 10, 2014:
http://dvbic.dcoe.mil/sites/default/files/u9/dod-tbi-worldwide-2000-2013Q1-as-of-130509.pdf

Department of Defense Directive 1332.18, "Separation or Retirement for Physical Disability," Washington, D.C., November 4, 1996, certified current as of December 1, 2003. As of January 10, 2014:
http://www.dtic.mil/whs/directives/corres/pdf/133218p.pdf

Department of Health and Human Services, *The HHS Poverty Guidelines for the Reminder of 2010*. August, 2010. As of June 19, 2013:
http://aspe.hhs.gov/poverty/10poverty.shtml

Dikmen, Sureyya, Joan Machamer, Bonnie Miller, Jason Doctor, and Nancy Temkin, "Functional Status Examination: A New Instrument for Assessing Outcome in

Traumatic Brain Injury," *Journal of Neurotrauma*, Vol. 18, No. 2, February 2001, pp. 127–140.

Dohrenwend, B. P., J. B. Turner, N. A. Turse, B. G. Adams, K. C. Koenen, and R. Marshall, "The Psychological Risks of Vietnam for U.S. Veterans: A Revisit with New Data and Methods," *Science*, Vol. 313, No. 5789, 2006, pp. 979–982. doi: 10.1126/science.1128944

Drake, Robert E., Gary R. Bond, and Deborah R. Becker, *Individual Placement and Support: An Evidence Support Based Approach to Supported Employment*, New York: Oxford University Press, 2012.

Dunn, Eric C., Nancy J. Wewiorski, and E. Sally Rogers, "The Meaning and Importance of Employment to People in Recovery from Serious Mental Illness: Results of a Qualitative Study," *Psychiatric Rehabilitation Journal*, Vol. 32, No. 1, 2008, pp. 59–62.

Elbogen, Eric B., Sally C. Johnson, H. Ryan Wagner, Virginia M. Newton, and Jean C. Beckham, "Financial Well-Being and Postdeployment Adjustment Among Iraq and Afghanistan War Veterans," *Military Medicine*, Vol. 177, No. 6, 2012, pp. 669–675.

Ettner, Susan L., Richard G. Frank, and Ronald C. Kessler, "The Impact of Psychiatric Disorders on Labor Market Outcomes," *Industrial and Labor Relations Review*, Vol. 51, No. 1, 1997.

Farrell, B. S., T. W. Gosling, S. E. Keisling, K. M. Nalwalk, S. Petrucci, and L. L. Shoemaker, *Military Personnel: Active Duty Benefits Reflect Changing Demographics, but Opportunities Exist to Improve*, Washington, D.C.: United States Government Accountability Office, 2002.

Feijo de Mello, M., J. de Jesus Mari, J. Bacaltchuk, H. Verdeli, and R. Neugebauer, "Systematic Review of Research Findings on the Efficacy of Interpersonal Therapy for Depressive Disorders," *European Archives of Psychiatry and Clinical Neuroscience*, Vol. 255, 2005, pp. 75–82.

Fischer, Hannah, *United States Military Casualty Statistics: Operation Iraqi Freedom and Operation Enduring Freedom*, Washington, D.C.: Congressional Research Service, Order Code RS22452, June 8, 2006. As of January 14, 2014: http://www.au.af.mil/au/awc/awcgate/crs/rs22452.pdf

Fouad, Nancy A., and John Bynner, "Work Transitions," *American Psychologist*, Vol. 63, No. 4, 2008, pp. 241–251.

Franklin, T. B., H. Russig, I. C. Weiss, J. Graff, N. Linder, A. Michalon, S. Vizi, and I. M. Mansuy, "Epigenetic Transmission of the Impact of Early Stress Across Generations," *Biological Psychiatry*, Vol. 68, No. 5, 2010, pp. 408–415.

Friedman, Matthew J., Patricia A. Resick, Richard A. Bryant, and Chris R. Brewin, "Considering PTSD for DSM-5," *Depression and Anxiety,* Volume 28, No. 9, September 2011, pp. 750–769. As of January 14, 2014: http://onlinelibrary.wiley.com/doi/10.1002/da.20767/pdf

GAO—*See* United States Government Accountability Office.

Grant, Bridget F., Frederick S. Stinson, Deborah A. Dawson, Patricia Chou, Mary C. Dufour, Wilson Compton, Roger P. Pickering, and Kenneth Kaplan, "Prevalence and Co-Occurrence of Substance Use Disorders and Independent Mood and Anxiety Disorders," *Archives of General Psychiatry*, Vol. 61, No. 8, 2004, pp. 807–816.

Grant, Jacqueline L., Eliver Eid Bou Ghosn, Robert C. Axtell, Katja Herges, Hedwich F. Kuipers, Nathan S. Woodling, Katrin Andreasson, Leonard A. Herzenberg, Leonore A. Herzenberg, and Lawrence Steinman, "Reversal of Paralysis and Reduced Inflammation from Peripheral Administration of β-Amyloid in TH1 and TH17 Versions of Experimental Autoimmune Encephalomyelitis," *Science Translational Medicine*, Vol. 4, No. 145, 2012, p. 145.

Graubard, B. I., and E. L. Korn, "Predictive Margins with Survey Data," *Biometrics*, Vol. 55, No. 2, 1999, pp. 652–659.

Grieger, Thomas A., Stephen J. Cozza, Robert J. Ursano, Charles Hoge, Patricia E. Martinez, Charles C. Engel, and Harold J. Wain, "Posttraumatic Stress Disorder and Depression in Battle-Injured Soldiers," *American Journal of Psychiatry*, Vol. 163, No. 10, October 2006, pp. 1777–1783.

Grill, Eric M., "'Care Beyond Duty'—The Air Force Wounded Warrior Program," May 2012. As of June 19, 2013: http://www.af.mil/news/story.asp?id=123301456

Guay, Stephane, Valerie Billette, and Andre Marchand, "Exploring the Links Between Posttraumatic Stress Disorder and Social Support: Processes and Potential Research Avenues," *Journal of Traumatic Stress*, Vol. 19, No. 3, 2006, pp. 327–338.

Hays, R. D., C. D. Sherbourne, and R. M. Mazel, "The RAND 36-Item Health Survey 1.0," *Health Economics*, Vol. 2, 1993, pp. 217–227.

Heaton, Paul, David S. Loughran, and Amalia R. Miller, *Compensating Wounded Warriors: An Analysis of Injury, Labor Market Earnings, and Disability Compensation Among Veterans of the Iraq and Afghanistan Wars*, Santa Monica,

Calif.: RAND Corporation, MG-1166-OSD, 2012. As of November 30, 2014:
http://www.rand.org/pubs/monographs/MG1166.html

Hogan, Brenda E., Wolfgang Linden, and Benjamin Najarian, "Social Support Interventions: Do They Work?" *Clinical Psychology Review*, Vol. 22, 2002, pp. 381–440.

Hoge, Charles W., Carl A. Castro, Stephen C. Messer, Dennis McGurk, Dave I. Cotting, and Robert L. Koffman, "Combat Duty in Iraq and Afghanistan, Mental Health Problems, Barriers to Care," *The New England Journal of Medicine*, Vol. 351, No. 1, 2004, pp. 13–22.

Hoge, C. W., D. McGurk, J. L. Thomas, A. L. Cox, C. C. Engel, and C. A. Castro, "Mild Traumatic Brain Injury in U.S. Soldiers Returning from Iraq," *The New England Journal of Medicine*, Vol. 358, 2008, pp. 453–463.

Hulin, Charles L., "Lessons From Industrial and Organizational Psychology," in Jeanne M. Brett and Fritz Drasgow, eds., *The Psychology of Work: Theoretically Based Empirical Research*, Mahwah, New Jersey: Lawrence Erlbaum Associates, 2002, pp. 3–22.

Institute of Medicine, *Broadening the Base of Treatment for Alcohol Problems*, Vol. 8, Washington, D.C.: National Academy Press, 1990.

Institute of Medicine of the National Academies, *Committee on Quality of Health in America: Improving the Quality of Health Care for Mental and Substance Use Conditions*, Washington, D.C.: The National Academies Press, 2006, pp. 77–139.

Institute of Medicine of the National Academies, "Returning Home from Iraq and Afghanistan Preliminary Assessment of Readjustment Needs of Veterans, Service Members, and Their Families," 2010. As of April 9, 2013:
http://www.nap.edu/catalog/12812.html

Institute of Medicine of the National Academies, "Treatment for Posttraumatic Stress Disorder in Military and Veteran Populations: Initial Assessment," 2012. As of June 19, 2013:
http://www.nap.edu/catalog.php?record_id=13364

IOM—*See* Institute of Medicine.

Jacobson, I. G., M. A. Ryan, T. I. Hooper, T. C. Smith, P. J. Amoroso, E. J. Boyko, G. D. Gackstetter, T. S. Wells, and N. S. Bell, "Alcohol Use and Alcohol-Related Problems Before and After Military Combat Deployment," *JAMA*, Vol. 300, No. 6, 2008, pp. 663–675.

Jennett, B., "Epidemiology of Head Injury," *Journal of Neurology, Neurosurgery, and Psychiatry,* Vol. 60, No. 3, 1996, pp. 62–69.

Jennett, B., "Epidemiology of Head Injury," *Archives of Disease in Childhood,* Vol. 78, 1998, pp. 403–406.

Joint Publication 1-02, *Department of Defense Dictionary of Military and Associated Terms,* Washington, D.C.: Joint Chiefs of Staff, November 8, 2010 (as amended through December 15, 2013). As of January 14, 2014:
http://www.dtic.mil/doctrine/new_pubs/jp1_02.pdf

Johnson, David R., "Assessing Marital Quality in Longitudinal and Life Course Studies," in J. C. Conoley and E. B. Werth, eds., *Family Assessment,* Lincoln, Neb.: Buros Institute of Mental Measurements, 1995, pp. 155–202.

Johnson, L., K. Mercer, D. Greenbaum, R. T. Bronson, D. Crowley, D. A. Tuveson, and T. Jacks, "Somatic Activation of the K-ras Oncogene Causes Early Onset Lung Cancer in Mice," *Nature,* Vol. 410, 2001, pp. 1111–1116.

Kanfer, Ruth, Connie R. Wanberg, and Tracy M. Kantrowitz, "Job Search and Employment: A Personality-Motivational Analysis and Meta-Analytic Review," *Journal of Applied Psychology,* Vol. 86, No. 5, 2001, pp. 837–855.

Kaniasty, Krzysztof, and Fran H. Norris, "Longitudinal Linkages Between Perceived Social Support and Posttraumatic Stress Symptoms: Sequential Roles of Social Causation and Social Selection," *Journal of Traumatic Stress,* Vol. 21, No. 3, June 2008, pp. 274–281.

Kehle, Shannon M., Melissa A. Polusny, Maureen Murdoch, Christopher R. Erbes, Paul A. Arbisi, Paul Thuras, and Laura A. Meis, "Early Mental Health Treatment-Seeking Among U.S. National Guard Soldiers Deployed to Iraq," *Journal of Traumatic Stress,* Vol. 23, 2010, pp. 33–40.

Kennedy, David P., Suzanne L. Wenzel, Ryan Brown, Joan S. Tucker, and Daniela Gilinelli, "Unprotected Sex Among Heterosexually Active Homeless Men: Results from a Multi-Level Dyadic Analysis," *AIDS and Behavior,* published online December 2, 2012. As of January 14, 2014:
http://rd.springer.com/article/10.1007%2Fs10461-012-0366-z/fulltext.html

Kessler, Ronald C., "Posttraumatic Stress Disorder: The Burden to the Individual and to Society," *Journal of Clinical Psychiatry,* Vol. 61, No. 5, 2000, pp. 4–14.

Kessler R. C., P. Berglund, O. Demler, R. Jin, D. Koretz, K. R. Meridangas, A. J. Rush, and P. S. Wang, "The Epidemiology of Major Depressive Disorder: Results from the

National Comorbidity Survey Replication (NCS-R)," *JAMA*, Vol. 289, No. 23, 2003, pp. 3095–3105.

Kessler, Ronald C., Wai Tat Chiu, Olga Demler, and Ellen E. Walters, "Prevalence, Severity, and Comorbidity of 12-Month DSM-IV Disorders in the National Comorbidity Survey Replication," *Archives of General Psychiatry*, Vol. 62, No. 6, June 2005, pp. 617–627.

Kessler, Ronald C., Amanda Sonnega, Evelyn Bromet, Michael Hughes, and Christopher B. Nelson, "Posttraumatic Stress Disorder in the National Comorbidity Survey," *Archives of General Psychiatry*, Vol. 52, 1995, pp. 1048–1060.

Kim P. Y., T. W. Britt, R. P. Klocko, L. A. Riviere, and A. Adler, "Stigma, Negative Attitudes About Treatment, and Utilization of Mental Health Care Among Soldiers," *Military Psychology*, Vol. 23, No. 1, 2011, pp. 65–81

Kirchner, JoAnn E., Mental Health QUERI Center Strategic Plan, North Little Rock, Ark.: Department of Veterans Affairs, Quality Enhancement Research Initiative (QUERI), 2011.

Kleykamp, Meredith, "Labor Market Outcomes Among Veterans and Military Spouses," in Janet M. Wilmoth and Andrew S. London, eds., *Life Course Perspectives on Military Service*, New York: Taylor and Francis, 2013, pp. 144–164.

Kleykamp, Meredith, "Unemployment, Earnings and Enrollment Among Post 9/11 Veterans," *Social Science Research*, Volume 42, Issue 3, May 2013, pp. 836–851. As of January 14, 2014:
http://www.sciencedirect.com/science/article/pii/S0049089X13000021#

Koegel, Paul, "Causes of Homelessness," *Encyclopedia of Homelessness*, Vol. 1, 2004, pp. 50–58.

Kraus, J. H., and S. B. Sorenson, "Epidemiology," in J. M. Silver, S. C. Yudofsky, and R. E. Hales, eds., *Neuropsychiatry of Traumatic Brain Injury*, Washington, D.C.: American Psychiatric Press, Inc., 1994, pp. 3–41.

Kroenke, Kurt, Robert L. Spitzer, and Janet B. W. Williams, "The PHQ-9: Validity of a Brief Depression Severity Measure," *Journal of General Internal Medicine,* Vol. 16, No. 9, September 2001, pp. 606–613.

Kuhn, Randall, and Dennis P. Culhane, "Applying Cluster Analysis to Test a Typology of Homelessness by Pattern of Shelter Utilization: Results from the Analysis of Administrative Data," *American Journal of Community Psychology*, Vol. 26, No. 2, April 1998, pp. 210–212.

Lara, M. E., and D. N. Klein, "Psychosocial Processes Underlying the Maintenance and Persistence of Depression: Implications for Understanding Chronic Depression," *Clinical Psychological Review*, Vol. 19, No. 5, 1999, pp. 553–570.

Lapierre, C. B., A. E. Schwegler, and B. J. LaBauve, "Posttraumatic Stress and Depression Symptoms in Soldiers Returning from Combat Operations in Iraq and Afghanistan," *Journal of Traumatic Stress*, Vol. 20, No. 6, 2007, pp. 933–943.

Leginski, Walter, "Historical and Contextual Influences on the U.S. Response to Contemporary Homelessness," March 2007. As of June 19, 2013: http://aspe.hhs.gov/hsp/homelessness/symposium07/leginski/

Loughran, David S., *Wage Growth in the Civilian Careers of Military Retirees,* Santa Monica, Calif.: RAND Corporation, MR-1363-OSD, 2002. As of January 14, 2014: http://www.rand.org/pubs/monograph_reports/MR1363.html

Löwe, Bernd, Kurt Kroenke, Wolfgang Herzog, and Kerstin Gräfe, "Measuring Depression Outcome with a Brief Self-Report Instrument: Sensitivity to Change of the Patient Health Questionnaire (PHQ-9)," *Journal of Affective Disorders*, Vol. 81, No. 1, July 2004, pp. 61–66.

Maguen, S., B. A. Lucenko, M. A. Reger, G. A. Gahm, B. T. Litz, K. H. Seal, Sara J. Knight, Charles R. Marmar, "The Impact of Reported Direct and Indirect Killing on Mental Health Symptoms in Iraq War Veterans," *Journal of Traumatic Stress*, Vol. 23, 2010, pp. 86–90.

The Management of MDD Working Group, "VA/DoD Clinical Practice Guideline for Management of Substance Use Disorders," Washington, D.C.: Department of Veterans Affairs, May 2009. As of June 19, 2013: http://www.healthquality.va.gov/mdd/mdd_full09_c.pdf

Marshall, B. D., M. R. Prescott, I. Liberzon, M. B. Tamburrino, J. R. Calabrese, and S. Galea, "Coincident Posttraumatic Stress Disorder and Depression Predict Alcohol Abuse During and After Deployment Among Army National Guard Soldiers," *Drug Alcohol Dependency*, Vol. 124, No. 3, 2012, pp. 193–199.

Mattiko, Mark J., Kristine L. Rae Olmsted, Janice M. Brown, and Robert M. Bray, "Alcohol Use and Negative Consequences Among Active Duty Military Personnel," *Addictive Behaviors*, Vol. 36, No. 6, 2011, pp. 608–614.

McKee-Ryan, Frances M., Zhaoli Song, Connie R. Wanberg, and Angelo J. Kinicki, "Psychological and Physical Well-Being During Unemployment: A Meta-Analytic Study," *Journal of Applied Psychology*, Vol. 90, No. 1, 2005, pp. 53–76.

Meis, Laura A., Christopher R. Erbes, Melissa A. Polusny, and Jill S. Compton, "Intimate Relationships Among Returning Soldiers: The Mediating and Moderating Roles of Negative Emotionality, PTSD Symptoms, and Alcohol Problems," *Journal of Traumatic Stress*, Vol. 23, No. 5, 2010, pp. 564–572. As of January 14, 2014: http://onlinelibrary.wiley.com/doi/10.1002/jts.20560/pdf

Mello, M. F., J. J. Mari, J. Bacaltchuk, H. Verdeli, and R. Neugebauer, "A Systematic Review of Research Findings on the Efficacy of Interpersonal Therapy for Depressive Disorders," *European Archives of Psychiatry and Clinical Neuroscience*, Vol. 255, 2005, pp. 75–82.

Miller, W. R., and P. L. Wilbourne, "Mesa Grande: A Methodological Analysis of Clinical Trials of Treatments for Alcohol Use Disorders," *Addiction,* Vol. 97, No. 3, 2000, pp. 265–277.

Milliken, Charles S., Jennifer L. Auchterlonie, and Charles W. Hoge, "Longitudinal Assessment of Mental Health Problems Among Active and Reserve Component Soldiers Returning from the Iraq War," *JAMA*, Vol. 298, No. 18, 2007, pp. 2141–2148.

Munsey, C., "Air Force Revitalizes Program that Matches Psychologists with Physicians," *American Psychological Association*, Vol. 40, No. 1, 2009, p. 13.

National Center for Injury Prevention and Control, *Traumatic Brain Injury in the United States: Emergency Department Visits, Hospitalizations and Deaths 2002–2006,* Washington, D.C.: U.S. Department of Health and Human Services, Centers for Disease Control and Prevention, March 2010. As of January 14, 2014: http://www.cdc.gov/traumaticbraininjury/pdf/blue_book.pdf

Newman, David J., Gordon M. Cragg, and Kenneth M. Snader, "Natural Products as Sources of New Drugs over the Period 1981–2002," *Journal of Natural Products,* Vol. 66, July 2003, pp. 1022–1037.

Nichols, Austin, Josh Mitchell, and Stephan Linder, *Consequences of Long-Term Unemployment*, Washington, D.C.: Urban Institute, 2013.

O'Connell, Maria J., Wesley Kasprow, and Robert A. Rosenheck, "Rates and Risk Factors for Homelessness after Successful Housing in a Sample of Formerly Homeless Veterans," *Psychiatric Services*, Vol. 59, No. 3, March 2008, pp. 268–275.

Olatunji, B. O., J. M. Cisler, and D. F. Tolin, "Qualify of Life in the Anxiety Disorders: A Meta-Analytic Review," *Clinical Psychology Review*, Vol. 27, 2007, pp. 572–581.

Olmsted, Kristine L. Rae, Janice M. Brown, J. Russ Vandermaas-Peeler, Stephen J. Tueller, Ruby E. Johnson, and Deborah A. Gibbs, "Mental Health and Substance

Abuse Treatment Stigma Among Soldiers," *Military Psychology*, Vol. 23, 2011, pp. 52–64.

Orcutt H. K., D. J. Erickson, and J. Wolfe, "The Course of PTSD Symptoms Among Gulf War Veterans: A Growth Mixture Modeling Approach," *Journal of Traumatic Stress*, Vol. 17, No. 3, 2004, pp. 195–202. doi: 10.1023/B:JOTS.0000029262.42865.c2

Ouellet, M. C., and C. M. Morin, "Efficacy of Cognitive-Behavioral Therapy for Insomnia Associated with Traumatic Brain Injury: A Single-Case Experimental Design," *Archives of Physical Medicine and Rehabilitation*, Vol. 88, No. 12, 2007, pp. 581–1592.

Ozer, Emily J., Suzanne R. Best, Tami L. Lipsey, and Daniel S. Weiss, "Predictors of Posttraumatic Stress Disorder and Symptoms in Adults: A Meta-Analysis," *Psychological Bulletin*, Vol. 129, No. 1, 2003, pp. 52–73.

Paniak C., G. Toller Lobe, A. Durand, and J. Nagy, "A Randomized Trial of Two Treatments for Mild Traumatic Brain Injury," *Brain Injury*, Vol. 12, No. 12, 1998, pp. 1011–1023.

Paniak C., G. Toller Lobe, S. Reynolds, A. Melnyk, J. Nagy, "A Randomized Trial of Two Treatments for Mild Traumatic Brain Injury: 1 Year Follow-Up," *Brain Injury*, Vol. 14, No. 3, 2000, pp. 219–226.

Payne D., S. P. Flaherty, M. F. Barry, and C. D. Mathews, "Preliminary Observations on Polar Body Extrusion and Pronuclear Formation in Human Oocytes Using Time Lapse Video Cinematography," *Human Reproduction*, Vol. 12, 1997, pp. 532–541.

Perl, Libby, *Veterans and Homelessness*, Washington, D.C.: Congressional Research Service, RL34024, April 1, 2011.

Perl, Libby, Erin Bagalman, Adrienne L. Fernandes-Alcantara, Elayne J. Heisler, Gail McCallion, and Francis X. McCarthy, *Homelessness: Targeted Federal Programs and Recent Legislation*, Washington, D.C.: Congressional Research Service, RL30442, May 17, 2012.

Peterson, Alan L., Cynthia A. Luethcke, Elisa V. Borah, Adam M. Borah, and Stacey Young-McCaughan, "Assessment and Treatment of Combat-Related PTSD in Returning War Veterans," *Journal of Clinical Psychology in Medical Settings*, Vol. 19, 2011, pp. 164–175. As of January 14, 2014: http://www.dtic.mil/dtic/tr/fulltext/u2/a558284.pdf

Ponsford, J., C. Willmott, A. Rothwell, P. Cameron, A-M Kelly, R. Nelms, and C. Curran, "Impact of Early Intervention on Outcome Following Mild Head Injury in Adults," *Journal of Neurology, Neurosurgery and Psychiatry,* Vol. 73, 2002,

pp. 330–332. As of January 14, 2014:
http://www.ncbi.nlm.nih.gov/pmc/articles/PMC1738009/pdf/v073p00330.pdf

President's New Freedom Commission on Mental Health, *Achieving the Promise: Transforming Mental Health Care in America*, Rockville, Md.: National Alliance on Mental Illness, 2003.

Price, Richard H., Amiram D. Vinokur, and Daniel S. Friedland, "The Job Seeker Role as Resource: Achieving Reemployment and Enhancing Mental Health," in Ann Maney and Juan Ramos, eds., *Socioeconomic Conditions, Stress and Mental Health Disorders: Toward a New Synthesis of Research and Public Policy*, Washington, D.C.: NIHM, 2002, pp. 1–27. As of January 14, 2014:
http://www.isr.umich.edu/src/seh/mprc/PDFs/The%20Job%20Seeker%20Role%20as%20Resource.pdf

Ramchand, Rajeev, Benjamin R. Karney, Karen Chan Osilla, Rachel M. Burns, and Leah Barnes Caldarone, "Prevalence of PTSD, Depression, and TBI Among Returning Servicemembers," in Terri Tanielian and Lisa H. Jaycox, eds., *Invisible Wounds of War: Psychological and Cognitive Injuries, Their Consequences, and Services to Assist Recovery,* Santa Monica, Calif.: RAND Corporation, MG-720-CCF, 2008, pp. 35–85. As of January 14, 2014:
http://www.rand.org/pubs/monographs/MG720.html

Ramchand, R., T. L. Schell, B. R. Karney, K. C. Osilla, R. M. Burns, and L. B. Caldarone, "Disparate Prevalence Estimates of PTSD Among Service Members Who Served in Iraq and Afghanistan: Possible Explanations," *Journal of Traumatic Stress*, Vol. 23, No. 1, 2010, pp. 59–68. doi: 10.1002/jts.20486

Rapaport, M. H., C. Clary, R. Fayyad, and J. Endicott, "Quality of Life Impairment in Depressive and Anxiety Disorders," *American Journal of Psychiatry*, Vol. 162, 2005, pp. 1171–1178.

Ren, Xinhua S., Katherine Skinner, Austin Lee, and Lewis Kazis, "Social Support, Social Selection and Self-Assessed Health Status: Results from the Veteran Health Study in the United States," *Social Science and Medicine*, Vol. 48, No. 12, 1999, pp. 1721–1734.

Resnick, Sandra G., Robert A. Rosenheck, and Charles E. Drebing, "What Makes Vocational Rehabilitation Effective? Program Characteristics Versus Employment Outcomes Nationally in VA," *Psychological Services*, Vol. 3, No. 4, 2006, pp. 239–248.

Rogers, J. M., and C. A. Read, "Psychiatric Comorbidity Following Traumatic Brain Injury," *Brain Injury*, Vol. 21, No. 13–14, 2007, pp. 1321–1333.

Rohling M. L., L. M. Binder, G. J. Demakis, G. J. Larrabee, D. M. Ploetz, and J. Langhinrichsen-Rohling, "A Meta-Analysis of Neuropsychological Outcome After Mild Traumatic Brain Injury: Re-Analyses and Reconsiderations of Binder et al. (1997), Frencham et al. (2005), and Pertab et al. (2009)," *The Clinical Neuropsychologist*, Vol. 25, 2011, pp. 608–623. As of January 14, 2014: http://www.ncbi.nlm.nih.gov/pubmed/21512956

Rona, R. J., M. Jones, J. Sundin, L. Goodwin, L. Hull, S. Wessely, and N. T. Fear, "Predicting Persistent Posttraumatic Stress Disorder (PTSD) in UK Military Personnel Who Served in Iraq: A Longitudinal Study," *Journal of Psychiatric Research*, Vol. 46, No. 9, 2012, pp. 1191–1198. doi: 10.1016/j.jpsychires.2012.05.009

Rosen, Craig S., Helen C. Chow, John F. Finney, Mark A. Greenbaum, Rudolf H. Moos, Javaid I. Sheikh, and Jerome A. Yesavage, "VA Practice Patterns and Practice Guidelines for Treating Posttraumatic Stress Disorder," *Journal of Traumatic Stress*, Vol. 17, No. 3, 2004, pp. 213–222.

Rosenheck, Robert, and Alan Fontana, "A Model of Homelessness Among Male Veterans of the Vietnam War Generation," *American Journal of Psychiatry*, Vol. 151, No. 3, 1994, pp. 421–427.

Ruffing, Kathy, "Testimony of Kathy A. Ruffing Senior Fellow, Center on Budget and Policy Priorities," testimony delivered to the Subcommittee on Social Security, Committee on Ways and Means, U.S. House of Representatives, Washington, D.C., August 9, 2013.

Ruzek, J. I., and R. C. Rosen, "Disseminating Evidence-Based Treatments for PTSD in Organizational Settings: A High Priority Focus Area," *Behaviour Research and Therapy*, Vol. 47, 2009, pp. 980–989.

Savoca, Elizabeth, and Robert Rosenheck, "The Civilian Labor Market Experiences of Vietnam-Era Veterans: The Influence of Psychiatric Disorders," *The Journal of Mental Health Policy and Economics*, Vol. 3, 2000, pp. 199–207.

Scarpello, Vida, and John P. Campbell, "Job Satisfaction: Are All Parts There?" *Personnel Psychology*, Vol. 36, No. 3, 1983, pp. 577–600.

Schell, Terry L., and Grant N. Marshall, "Survey of Individuals Previously Deployed for OEF/OIF," in Terri Tanielian and Lisa H. Jaycox, eds., *Invisible Wounds of War: Psychological and Cognitive Injuries, Their Consequences, and Services to Assist Recovery*, Santa Monica, Calif.: RAND Corporation, MG-720-CCF, 2008, pp. 87–115. As of January 14, 2014: http://www.rand.org/pubs/monographs/MG720z1.html

Schnurr, P. P., A. F. Hayes, C. A. Lunney, M. McFall, and M. Uddo, "Longitudinal Analysis of the Relationship Between Symptoms and Quality of Life in Veterans Treated for Posttraumatic Stress Disorder," *Journal of Consulting and Clinical Psychology*, Vol. 74, No. 4, August 2006, pp. 707–713.

Schell, T. L., G. N. Marshall, and L. H. Jaycox, "All Symptoms Are Not Created Equal: The Prominent Role of Hyperarousal in the Natural Course of Posttraumatic Psychological Distress," *Journal of Abnormal Psychology*, Vol. 113, No. 2, 2004, pp. 189–197. doi: 10.1037/0021-843X.113.2.189

Schultz, A. B., and D. W. Edington, "Analysis of the Association Between Metabolic Syndrome and Disease in a Workplace Population Over Time," *Value in Health: The Journal of the International Society for Pharmacoeconomics and Outcomes Research*, Vol. 13, No. 2, March–April 2010, pp. 258–264.

Schwab, C. G., S. E. Boucher, and B. K. Sloan, "Metabolizable Protein and Amino Acid Nutrition of the Cow: Where Are We in 2007?" *Proclamation of the 68th Annual Minnesota Nutrition Conference*, 2007, pp. 121–138.

Schwab, R., J. F. Palatnik, M. Riester, C. Schommer, M. Schmid, and D. Weigel, "Specific Effects of MicroRNAs on the Plant Transcriptome," *Developmental Cell*, Vol. 8, April 2005, pp. 517–527.

Seal, K. H., G. Cohen, A. Waldrop, B. E. Cohen, S. Maguen, and L. Ren, "Substance Use Disorders in Iraq and Afghanistan Veterans in VA Healthcare, 2001–2010: Implications for Screening, Diagnosis, and Treatment," *Drug and Alcohol Dependence*, Vol. 116, No. 1, 2011, pp. 93–101.

Setodji, C. M., M. Scheuner, J. S. Pankow, R. S. Blumenthal, H. Chen, and E. Keeler, "A Graphical Method for Assessing Risk Factor Threshold Values Using the Generalized Additive Model: The Multi-Ethnic Study of Atherosclerosis," *Health Services and Outcomes Research Methodology*, Vol. 12, No. 1, 2012, pp. 62–79. doi: 10.1007/s10742-012-0082-1

Shafrana, R., D. M. Clark, C. G. Fairburne, A. Arntz, D. H. Barlow, A. Ehlers, M. Freeston, P. A. Garety, S. D. Hollon, L. G. Ost, P. M. Salkovskis, J. M. G. Williams, and G. T. Wilson, "Mind the Gap: Improving the Dissemination of CBT," *Behaviour Research and Therapy*, Vol. 47, 2009, pp. 902–909.

Shalev, A. Y., S. Freedman, T. Peri, D. Brandes, T. Sahar, S. P. Orr, and R. K. Pitman, "Prospective Study of Posttraumatic Stress Disorder and Depression Following Trauma," *American Journal of Psychiatry*, Vol. 155, No. 5, 1998, pp. 630–637.

Shanahan, Michael J., "Pathways to Adulthood in Changing Societies: Variability and Mechanisms in Life Course Perspective," *Annual Review of Sociology*, Vol. 26, 2000, pp. 667–692.

Shen, Yu-Chu, Jeremy Arkes, and Thomas V. Williams, "Effects of Iraq/Afghanistan Deployments on Major Depression and Substance Use Disorder: Analysis of Active Duty Personnel in the US Military," *American Journal of Public Health*, Vol. 102, No. S1, 2012, pp. S80–S87.

Sherman, Michelle D., Dona K. Zanotti, and Dan E. Jones, "Key Elements in Couples Therapy with Veterans with Combat-Related Posttraumatic Stress Disorder," *Professional Psychology: Research and Practice*, Vol. 36, No. 6, 2005, pp. 626–633.

Sloan, D. M., B. P. Marx, and T. M. Keane, "Reducing the Burden of Mental Illness in Military Veterans: Commentary on Kazdin and Blasé," *Perspectives on Psychological Science*, Vol. 6, 2011, pp. 503–506.

Smith, Besa, Margaret A. K. Ryan, Deborah L. Wingard, Thomas L. Patterson, Donald J. Slymen, and Caroline A. Macera, for the Millennium Cohort Study Team, "Cigarette Smoking and Military Deployment: A Prospective Evaluation," *American Journal of Preventive Medicine*, Vol. 35, No. 6, 2008, pp. 539–546.

Smith, M. W., P. P. Schnurr, R. A. Rosenheck, M. W. Smith, "Employment Outcomes and PTSD Symptom Severity," *Mental Health Services Research*, Vol. 7, No. 2, 2005, pp. 89–101.

Smith, T. C., M. A. Ryan, D. L. Wingard, D. J. Slymen, J. F. Sallis, D. Kritz-Silverstein, and Millennium Cohort Study Team, "New Onset and Persistent Symptoms of Post-Traumatic Stress Disorder Self Reported After Deployment and Combat Exposures: Prospective Population Based US Military Cohort Study," *BMJ*, Vol. 336, No. 7640, 2008, pp. 366–371. doi: 10.1136/bmj.39430.638241.AE

Southwick, S. M., C. A. Morgan III, A. Darnell, D. Bremner, A. L. Nicolaou, L. M. Nagy, and D. S. Charney, "Trauma-Related Symptoms in Veterans of Operation Desert Storm: A 2-Year Follow-Up," *American Journal of Psychiatry*, Vol. 152, No. 8, 1995, pp. 1150–1155.

Spera, Christopher, Randall K. Thomas, Frances Barlas, Ronald Szoc, and Milton H. Cambridge, "Relationship of Military Deployment Recency, Frequency, Duration, and Combat Exposure to Alcohol Use in the Air Force," *Journal of Studies on Alcohol and Drugs*, Vol. 72, No. 1, January 2011, pp. 5–14. As of January 14, 2014: http://www.jsad.com/jsad/downloadarticle/Relationship_of_Military_Deployment_Recency_Frequency_Duration_and_Comba/4844.pdf

Stansfeld, S. A., R. Roberts, and S. Foot, "Assessing the Validity of the SF-36 General Health Survey," *Quality of Life Research*, Vol. 6, 1997, pp. 217–224.

Starr, L. R., and J. Davila, "Excessive Reassurance Seeking, Depression, and Interpersonal Rejection: A Meta-Analytic Review," *Journal of Abnormal Psychology*, Vol. 117, 2008, pp. 762–775.

Sundin, J., N. T. Fear, A. Iversen, R. J. Rona, and S. Wessely, "PTSD After Deployment to Iraq: Conflicting Rates, Conflicting Claims," *Psychological Medicine*, Vol. 40, No. 3, 2010, pp. 367–382. doi: 10.1017/S0033291709990791

Suris, A., and L. Lind, "Military Sexual Trauma: A Review of Prevalence and Associated Health Consequences in Veterans," *Trauma, Violence, and Abuse*, Vol. 9, No. 4, 2008, pp. 250–269. doi: 10.1177/1524838008324419

Tanielian, Terri, and Lisa H. Jaycox, eds., *Invisible Wounds of War: Psychological and Cognitive Injuries, Their Consequences, and Services to Assist Recovery*, Santa Monica, Calif.: RAND Corporation, MG-720-CCF, 2008. As of January 14, 2014: http://www.rand.org/pubs/monographs/MG720.html

Thoits, Peggy A., "Conceptual, Methodological, and Theoretical Problems in Studying Social Support as a Buffer Against Life Stress," *Journal of Health and Social Behavior*, Vol. 23, No. 2, 1982, pp. 145–159.

Thomas, Jeffrey L., Joshua E. Wilk, Lyndon A. Riviere, Dennis McGurk, Carl A. Castro, and Charles W. Hoge, "Prevalence of Mental Health Problems and Functional Impairment Among Active Component and National Guard Soldiers 3 and 12 Months Following Combat in Iraq," *Archives of General Psychiatry*, Vol. 67, No. 6, 2010, pp. 614–623.

United States Government Accountability Office, *Employment for People with Disabilities: Little is Known about the Effectiveness of Fragmented and Overlapping Programs*, Washington, D.C., GAO-12-677, June 29, 2012. As of January 14, 2014: http://www.gao.gov/products/GAO-12-677

U.S. Department of Defense, *Annual Report to Congress on Plans for the Department of Defense for the Support of Military Family Readiness*, Washington, D.C., 2012.

U.S. Department of Defense, *Annual Report to the Congressional Defense Committees on the Department of Defense Military Family Readiness Council*, Washington, D.C., 2012.

Vasterling, J. J., M. Verfaellie, and K. D. Sullivan, "Mild Traumatic Brain Injury and Posttraumatic Stress Disorder in Returning Veterans: Perspectives from Cognitive Neuroscience," *Clinical Psychology Review*, Vol. 29, No. 8, 2009, pp. 674–684.

Vaughan, Christine Anne, Terry L. Schell, Lisa H. Jaycox, Grant N. Marshall, and Terri Tanielian, "Quantitative Needs Assessment of New York State Veterans and Their Spouses," in Terry L. Schell and Terri Tanielian, eds., *A Needs Assessment of New York State Veterans: Final Report to the New York State Health Foundation,* Santa Monica, Calif.: RAND Corporation, TR-920-NYSHF, 2011, pp. 23–49. As of January 14, 2014:
http://www.rand.org/pubs/technical_reports/TR920.html.html

Vinokur, Amiram, Robert D. Caplan, and Cindy C. Williams, "Effects of Recent and Past Stress on Mental Health: Coping with Unemployment Among Vietnam Veterans and Nonveterans," *Journal of Applied Social Psychology*, Vol. 17, Issue 8, 1987, pp. 710–730.

Vinokur, A. D., R. H. Price, and R. D. Caplan, "From Field Experiments to Program Implementation: Assessing the Potential Outcomes of an Experimental Intervention Program for Unemployed Persons," *American Journal of Community Psychology,* Vol. 19, No. 4, 1991, pp. 543–562.

Vinokur, A. D., R. H. Price, and Y. Schul, "Impact of the JOBS Intervention on Unemployed Workers Varying in Risk for Depression," *American Journal of Community Psychology*, Vol. 23, 1995, pp. 39–74.

Vogt, Dawne, "Mental Health-Related Beliefs as a Barrier to Service Use for Military Personnel and Veterans: A Review," *Psychiatric Services*, Vol. 62, No. 2, 1999, pp. 135–142.

Wade, D. T., S. Crawford, F. J. Wenden, S. Crawford, and F.E. Caldwell, "Does Routine Follow-Up After Head Injury Help? A Randomised Controlled Trial," *Journal of Neurology, Neurosurgery and Psychiatry*, Vol. 62, 1997, pp. 478–484.

Wade, D. T., N. S. King, F. J. Wenden, S. Crawford, and F.E. Caldwell, "Routine Follow-Up After Head Injury: A Second Randomized Controlled Trial," *Journal of Neurology, Neurosurgery and Psychiatry*, Vol. 65, 1998, pp. 177–83.

Wanberg, Connie R., "The Individual Experience of Unemployment," *Annual Review of Psychology*, Vol. 63, 2012, pp. 369–396.

Warden, Deborah, "Military TBI During the Iraq and Afghanistan Wars," *Journal of Head Trauma Rehabilitation*, Vol. 21, No. 5, 2006, pp. 398–402.

Warden, Deborah L., Barry Gordon, Thomas W. McAllister, Jonathan M. Silver, Jeffery T. Barth, John Bruns, Angela Drake, Tony Gentry, Andy Jagoda, Douglas I. Katz, Jess Kraus, Lawrence A. Labbate, Laurie M. Ryan, Molly B. Sparling, Beverly Walters, John Whyte, Ashley Zapata, and George Zitnay, "Guidelines for the Pharmacologic Treatment of Neurobehavioral Sequelae of Traumatic Brain Injury,"

Journal of Neurotrauma, Vol. 23, No. 10, October 2006, pp. 1468–1501. As of January 14, 2014:
http://www.ncbi.nlm.nih.gov/pubmed/17020483

Ware, John E., Kristin K. Snow, Mark Kosinski, and Barbara Gandek, *SF-36 Health Survey: Manual and Interpretation Guide*, Boston, Mass.: Health Institute, New England Medical Center, 1993.

Warner, Christopher H., George N. Appenzeller, Thomas Grieger, Slava Belenkiy, Jill Breitbach, Jessica Parker, Carolynn M. Warner, and Charles Hoge, "Importance of Anonymity to Encourage Honest Reporting in Mental Health Screening After Combat Deployment," *Archives of General Psychiatry*, Vol. 68, No. 10, 2011, pp. 1065–1071.

Warr, Peter, John Cook, and Toby Wall, "Scales for the Measurement of Some Work Attitudes and Aspects of Psychological Well-Being," *Journal of Occupational Psychology*, Vol. 52, 1979, pp. 129–148.

Warr, Peter, Paul Jackson, and Michael Banks, "Unemployment and Mental Health: Some British Studies," *Journal of Social Issues*, Vol. 44, No. 4, 1998, pp. 47–68.

Watkins, K. E., H. A. Pincus, S. Paddock, B. Smith, A. Woodroffe, C. Farmer, M. E. Sorbero, M. Horvitz-Lennon, T. Mannle, K. A. Hepner, J. Solomon, and C. Call, "Care for Veterans with Mental and Substance Use Disorders: Good Performance but Room to Improve on Many Measures," *Health Affairs*, Vol. 30, No. 11, 2011, pp. 2194–2203.

Weathers, F., J. Huska, and T. Keane, *The PTSD Checklist Military Version (PCL-M),* Boston, Mass.: National Center for PTSD, 1991.

Weathers, F. W., B. T. Litz, D. S. Herman, J. A. Huska, and T. M. Keane, "The PTSD Checklist (PCL): Reliability, Validity, and Diagnostic Utility," paper presented at the International Society for Traumatic Stress Studies, San Antonio, Texas, 1993.

Weinick, Robin M., Ellen Burke Beckjord, Carrie M. Farmer, Laurie T. Martin, Emily M. Gillen, Joie Acosta, Michael P. Fisher, Jeffrey Garnett, Gabriella C. Gonzalez, Todd C. Helmus, Lisa H. Jaycox, Kerry Reynolds, Nicholas Salcedo, and Deborah M. Scharf, *Programs Addressing Psychological Health and Traumatic Brain Injury Among U.S. Military Servicemembers and Their Families,* Santa Monica, Calif.: RAND Corporation, TR-950-OSD. As of June 19, 2013:
http://www.rand.org/pubs/technical_reports/TR950.html

Weiss, R., G. Dawis, G. England, and L. Lofquist, *Minnesota Studies in Vocational Rehabilitation 22: Manual for the Minnesota Satisfaction Questionnaire,* Minneapolis: University of Minnesota, 1967.

Wells, Timothy, Cynthia Leard Mann, Sarah Fortuna, Besa Smith, Tyler C. Smith, Margaret A. K. Ryan, Edward J. Boyko, and Dan Blazer, "A Prospective Study of Depression Following Combat Deployment in Support of the Wars in Iraq and Afghanistan," *American Journal of Public Health*, Vol. 100, No. 1, 2010, pp. 90–99.

Wells, Timothy S., Shannon C. Miller, Amy B. Adler, Charles C. Engel, Tyler C. Smith, and John A. Fairbank, *Mental Health Impact of the Iraq and Afghanistan Conflicts: A Review of U.S. Research, Service Provision, and Programmatic Responses*, San Diego, Calif.: Naval Health Research Center, Report No. 11-10, 2011.

Wenzel, S. L., *Alcohol Use and HIV Risk Among Impoverished Women*, Rockville, Md.: National Institute on Alcohol Abuse and Alcoholism, 2005.

Wills, Thomas A., and Ori Shinar, "Measuring Perceived and Received Social Support," in Sheldon Cohen, Lynn G. Underwood, and Benjamin H. Gottlieb, eds., *Social Support Measurement and Intervention*, New York: Oxford University Press, 2000, pp. 86–135.

Zatzick, D. F., C. R. Marmar, D. S. Weiss, W. S. Browner, T. J. Metzler, J. M. Golding, A. Stewart, W. E. Schlenger, and K. B. Wells, "Posttraumatic Stress Disorder and Functioning and Quality of Life in a Nationally Representative Sample of Male Vietnam Veterans," *American Journal of Psychiatry*, Vol. 154, 1997, pp. 1690–1695.